Introduction to the Submissive Lifestyle and Thrilling BDSM Experiences

Alexandra Morris

Hey,

Thank you very much for choosing this book!

Before we begin...

If you are interested in non-fiction sex books, head over to our partner site alexandramorris.com

Alexandramorris.com is a great site in the making. They publish e-books, paperbacks, audiobooks and blog posts written by up-and-coming writers and great freelancers. They also give away TONS of Audible coupon codes, Amazon gift cards, pdf copies of books totally free!

We really hope this books will give you valuable information to take your sex life to the next level. Enjoy and please leave an honest review after finishing it.

Best regards

Table of Contents

PART ONE

The Submissive Role

Chapter One: Introduction 3

Chapter Two: Describing the Submissive 21

    Service Submission 22

    Sex Submission 25

    Pain Submissives...31

Chapter Three: Subcultures...77

    The Slave 77

    Pet 81

    Little...87

Sissy maid.. 89

Brat.. 91

PART TWO

Building a Great Submissive Relationship

Chapter Four: Principles of a Healthy Relationship...... 105

PART THREE

Action Plans

Chapter Five: Getting Started with the Lifestyle........... 119

Chapter Six: Now that You've Found a Partner............ 125

Chapter Seven: Ideas to Try.. 129

Role Play 129

Bondage 144

Talk 148

Asking Permission 149

Punishments..152

The Pain Factor 154

Sex Toys..156

Expanding to Outside the Bedroom.............158

Human Ashtray..162

Conclusion: Tips to Remember 177

References...181

BONUS

Preview of Dominant Women: The Dominant Women's and Submissive Men's Handbook For Amazing Relationships

Introduction..185

PART ONE: BEING A DOMINANT WOMAN 191

Start Slowly 194

Different Ways of Being a Domme..............................216

Financial...222

Household Chores..224

Childcare..226

Different Measures of Success 228

PART ONE

The Submissive Role

CHAPTER ONE
Introduction

Many regard the role of being a submissive as perverse or outside the realms of what larger society perceives as normal sex. However, this judgment is perhaps made on the basis of too little knowledge of how truly rewarding adopting the stance of the sub can be. It is probably more generally acceptable for the male to be in a dominant role and the female to be the submissive. This is easy to understand bearing in mind the constraints which society imposes upon us all and how we are all shaped by our experiences.

During World War II, and indeed every other war, men disappeared from the workforce and women had to step up to the plate and take their place in the labor market. Understandably, they became more macho and were responsible for putting food on the table for their families. At the end of the war, when men returned and stepped back into the world of business, trade and commerce, women were encouraged to retake their place in the home. Even fashion reflected the role, which was expected of them. Dresses emphasized their small waists and they began to remove the overalls they wore in the factories of the war and replace them with feminine styles, and paint their faces to look as appealing to men as they could. Man became the master of his own castle again.

In the 1950's their lives became easier with the influx of new domestic appliances and women appeared on TV enthusing wildly because they now possessed an electric vacuum cleaner. This meant they had more time to spend on making themselves look pretty for when their husbands got home. Women were there to be sexually available to their hardworking mates who provided for them and thus had the privilege of dictating their wives' life in almost all areas. If we look at ads that appeared in newspapers or magazines in the 1950's now, it seems impossible that the world has changed so much and that the roles of men and women have found a level where they are both much more in balance. This imbalance of the sexes was portrayed in films where the little woman would not obey her master was forced over his knee and spanked, as she screamed and kicked her legs shouting that she wanted to be free. He would then release her and kiss her passionately, a kiss that she would gratefully receive and return.

In the 1960's, with the advent of the contraceptive pill, which controlled the woman's menstrual cycle and gave her the power to decide when and if to have children, this shifted even more so, with women burning their metaphorical bras, demanding equality in all areas, including sexual freedom. Some said that the pill gives license to promiscuity but that meant that while it was okay for men to sleep around. If a woman did the same thing she was regarded as a slut. It could be argued that many women missed the point altogether because the freedom they had desired actually resulted in them having to take on more responsibility for not many more benefits than they'd started with.

The clever ones were the ones who took what they wanted from all the best bits. They could still agree to be the little lady at home and take advantage of the way that the woman's role in society, in general, was changing. They could still be treated to meals out; all their clothes were bought and paid for by their husbands, their hairdos were paid for, holidays, social events; provided their husband had a good enough salary, then these were still in abundance. These women still received all this and the only thing they had to trade was doing the housework, looking after the children and having sex. And now that sex had been revolutionized for women so that they realized it was something that they should have been enjoying all along, and that they could ask for what they wanted sexually, the women at home began to have it much easier than those who had fought for equal rights and said that they preferred to work rather than stay at home. If they were really clever, they worked out how to have an extremely satisfying sex life and get their husband to do the housework too – or at least help her. All it took was a little careful persuasion and the promise of fantastic sex. They were propagating the idea and practice of a submissive/dominant relationship and it was suitable for both parties. This had evolved from the needs of the economy and as the economy changed again, then so too did the role of the people who were responsible for upholding it and making it work.

Now, working women found themselves in employment and doing everything the women at home did too. Much to the working woman's dismay, she found that her rights were not equal to that of a man and nor was her salary. She was – and still is in many occupations – receiving far less for doing the same job as her male counterpart. Shirley Conran even wrote a book in 1975 about this called Superwoman because a woman was expected to be all things to all people at all times. If you were to pick up a copy now, the household tips she gave to the then modern woman would be laughed at because it serves as a perfect example of how gender roles have changed over those few short decades.

Another Shirley who brought this point home was Shirley Valentine who felt so taken for granted she decided to stay in Greece at the end of her girly holiday. She hadn't even told her husband that she was going and used to talk to the walls because those were the only things that didn't answer back. When her husband came home and found the note on the table, he could not believe his eyes. She had been such a devoted little wife and mother, also abused by her teenage daughter who used her like a slave. So she got a job in a bar in Greece and had a quick sex fling with a Greek who told her she was beautiful. She believed him for however such a brief amount of time, until she caught him giving the same spiel to another woman off the next plane. Finally, her husband arrived, realizing that he couldn't live without her. When he arrived, she was sitting at the edge of the sea sipping a glass of Retsina and she had changed so much that he walked past her without recognition, carrying his little suitcase and wearing his best suit. But she didn't just change on the outside. Everything in her world had changed too because she held her hand up and said, "Enough! I'm worth so much more than this." You were left not knowing if she went back with him, but you hoped that if she did, she would never relinquish that power she had just earned for herself. And that was what it was like for the '60's and '70's woman. Freedom had been hard fought for and Shirley Valentine had shown them how easy it was to change your life for good. All it took was one brave step into the wilderness to come back stronger and more independent. If she could gather up that courage, then the new woman had all the power she needed to step into her new role as dominant or, at the very least, equal.

With the advent of the late 1970's/early 1980's, technology was just beginning to show its head and everyone in the workforce began to feel its ripples in their lives, specifically in their working lives. As it gathered momentum, the whole appearance of the commercial world began to be shaken up. Industry was increasingly being done by machines and what had traditionally been the domain of the working man became obsolete and defunct, and huge swathes of the male workforce became surplus to requirements, seemingly overnight. Men who had been dependent on their jobs as defining who they were, floundered, no longer sure of what or who they were supposed to be.

Significantly more women entered higher education and graduated from universities into high-powered and well paying jobs. It began to dawn on them that men might indeed be superfluous to their lifestyles, certainly financially, and that the only thing that they might need them for was sex. Many women began to feel more dominant and this expanded into many couples' sex lives. However, human beings are social animals and although the institution of marriage began to break down with a massive increase in divorce rates, people still came together to cohabitate and raise children within a secure and stable household.

Women began to take control of their sex lives and demanded what they wanted in bed. A wave of liberation blew through the land, although homosexuality was still not legalized in America until 2003, it could clearly be felt that the times really were changing. Women became more aggressive in asking for what they wanted sexually and some men willingly obliged relishing being told what to do by a sexy, confident woman who knew what she wanted and how to get it. Women were used to having it the other way, with the man dictating what he wanted. Many tolerated poor sex when the man would take what he wanted before falling asleep, leaving his partner unsatisfied and unfulfilled. The sexual revolution gave women the key to release themselves and take the reins to ride to a better sexual future.

As sexual practices became more visible and accessible in women's magazines such as Cosmopolitan, and the media generally, certainly in the western world, exposed sexual practices to a new generation they could only ever have dreamed about. Sex came into the public arena much more forcibly. They began to introduce things into their own sex lives that their mothers and grandmothers would have blushed at, and launched themselves into a world that continued to open up before them to offer pleasure they had to not previously experienced. They were no longer willing to submit to sexless, loveless sex that left them discontent and wanting more, far more. Not surprisingly, their partners welcomed the new adventures that were being offered to them and were reeled into compliance so that they could benefit from the new sexual revolution.

Numerous different sexual proclivities became as well known and talked about as often as what people were having for dinner. People's attitudes began to relax around the subject as it was openly discussed in the still developing new sexual revolution. Boundaries around sexuality relaxed and women were encouraged by numerous publications and women's lib movements to go for what they wanted. The trouble was that they were used to being the underdog and being taken for granted, and many decided to turn the tables on the man who had made his demands felt and had them met, usually because women felt they had no choice. But now they had. There was no reason now for them not to ask for what they wanted and be confident that they would receive it.

Needless to say, many men enjoyed the sexual freedom that women found too. It meant that they didn't have to do all the work when it came to sex. More often than not, they enjoyed women taking the initiative and demanding sex. It turned them on so complying with their woman's wishes was no big deal. As women's sexual confidence grew, they began to demand more and more. They read about their G Spot and began to insist that they partner search for it thoroughly. They wanted more than a quick wham bam, thank you ma'am, and wanted to experiment and play out their fantasies. This could include being spanked themselves, which the male quite often relished, but it could also for some demand that they be allowed to spank the male instead. This corporal punishment could also extend into being tied up, blindfolded, gagged, hair pulling, rough sex but it could also be meted out by the female on the male.

The BDSM (Bondage, Domination, Sadism and Masochism) movement was well and truly born into a modern western world, a world where almost anything became acceptable. People who shared this kind of sex life became more vocal and visible, unashamed of who they were and what they wanted. Clubs sprang up to cater specifically for this sexual proclivity.

However, some still struggled with this new freedom. After all, guilt came alongside the desire to step outside the boundaries so carefully and thoroughly introduced to us from birth to stick to healthy and wholesome natural and normal sex. But, of course, it depends on the definition of normalcy and as more and more people wrestled with this concept, the boundaries were pushed and people felt encouraged to question their doubts in an effort to become more fulfilled sexually. Most were fed up with vanilla sex and boredom in the bedroom, and with the promise of adventurous and exciting sex being pushed at them from all quarters, they began to gather more knowledge and question how they could get it too.

Couples who had always been led to believe that BDSM was weird or perverted discovered that this was not the case at all. They found that in fact, it provided a bond more profound than they had ever known because they were trusting another human being with not just their bodies but with their complete welfare. Adopting this lifestyle was not always an easy thing to do though because of all the baggage they carried from their childhoods. Having a loving partner to expound their innermost thoughts and fears demanded that they were more honest, not only to another person but themselves too. It helped people to explore their own psyches and understand how and why they might carry misconceptions that prevented them from leading full and satisfying sex lives.

An increasing number of people sought CBT (on this occasion Cognitive Behavior Therapy - not cock and ball torture) as they started to follow the path to self discovery. They began to question why they felt the way they did and with new self knowledge they moved on, ridding themselves of misguided guilt and inhibitions that had grown too heavy.

Allowing someone to perform potentially painful practices on their bodies meant that they had to put their trust in someone else. They handed over their own power to someone else. Certainly, for the older generation who could still remember strong gender-defined divisions, this was a huge leap of faith. However, they found that when they started along this path, their lives were changed for the better. They rekindled a passion that they may have lost along the way and felt complicit in a secret that up to now a proportionally small number were privy to.

Pop culture propagated the fact that BDSM was normal and could add a hitherto much maligned forbidden pleasure to everyone's sex lives. Films such as Fifty Shades of Grey became box office hits and this trilogy of books on BDSM titillated the western world and became best sellers. It would seem that this type of sex might not be as distasteful and repugnant as we had been led to believe. BDSM is now infiltrating society at all levels and is losing its bad reputation. Sex shops are becoming more visible and instead of having blacked out windows, softer sex shops are springing up in abundance selling sex toys and women hold sex aid parties where there is much wine normally imbibed, much giggling but many sales made.

And why shouldn't there be giggling? Why should sex be serious? Sex is something that we should be enjoying in all its glory, and if two people agree to it, then how can it be wrong? As long as it is hurting no one else, then drop those inhibitions and enter a world that could rock your foundations and change life as you've known it forever. Dismiss those groundless, outdated ideas that you are being asked to commit to a life of sex slavery and that it is cold sex at its most base level. BDSM can be a magical wonderland where two people commit to each other at the most fundamental level and make a deeper connection than they may have ever thought possible. Try to bear in mind that wonderful phrase which says it all: Don't knock it until you've tried it. You will be sorry that you have not done this before. It is such a powerful a tool that it could save a failing relationship, pep up a boring one and bring two people closer together than they ever thought possible.

CHAPTER TWO
Describing the Submissive

S ubmission is not a homogenous thing that looks the same for everyone. Each relationship is different just like in non-Dom/Sub relationships. Submission has many faces and forms and the only common thread being that there needs to be trust with the Dominant. Using broad strokes, the types of Submission can be named as:

- Service

- Sexual

- Pain

- Some combination of the above.

Service Submission

The first thing a Submissive focuses on when identifying as such as their need to be of service. This could range from sex and play to more mundane activities. Service involves activities that ease the life of the Dominant partner. This could range from making his first fortifying cup of coffee in the morning to laying out his work clothes to doing daily chores. Of course, play and sex also comes into it but that is just one aspect of the relationship. A Domestic Submissive for example has a completely different idea of what service means than a service Submissive.

They both feel contented and happy when they serve their Dominant but what that service looks like could be very different. A Domestic Submissive generally does not have much sexual interaction with their owner. They take pleasure in cleaning for others.

Therefore, how can we define what it is to be of service to your Dominant? Does it encompass everything from doing chores around the house to looking after pets and family? Maybe paying the household bills and running all the errands? Is it doing the job of a personal assistant and keeping the Dominant on schedule for everything that has to be done? Organizing their life to their satisfaction? Or is it being a sex object that seeks to fulfill every fantasy the Dominant has ever had? Cater to their every whim? The answer is that all of these fall under the umbrella of service Submissive. It has a wide spectrum of duties and responsibilities that fall under the service purview such as cooking, grooming, personal training, event planning, home repair, child care, cleaning, pet care, chauffeuring, secretarial duties or even just providing intellectual conversation.

For the Submissive, discovering where they fit in the service spectrum is not a simple thing. They have to identify their desires and needs in a relationship first and then choose those aspects of service that cater to them. If what the Submissive needs is structure, they would need a home control journal to get started. This is simply a journal which enables you to plan your activities as pertains to keeping a home functioning at optimum conditions.

Should you wish to focus on sexual services skills, it is possible to do so in various ways. It all depends on what you want.

Service Submissives derive joy and happiness from being asked to do the most menial of tasks. It is not just the sexual services that apply here as it can also encompass domestic duties, administrative duties and chauffeuring among other things.

This kind of Submissive is special because they have the ability to adjust to any type of service their Dominant might require of them with very little training. They are very rare and unique types of people and this type of Submissive is not for everyone. This is because they can perform well as a personal assistant, answering phones, keeping up with correspondence, managing the schedule and making sure the Dominant stays hydrated. Or they could be a body servant who bathes, shaves, grooms and generally oversees the health and wellness of the Dom. Or the service Submissive could be an escort or social elitist who charms the Dom's friends and reflects well on them as a partner. If the Dom is a masochist, the service Sub might have to learn to play games which service the Dom.

Sex Submission

As we have seen, BDSM consists of more than rough sex among consenting individuals. There needs to be established trust mentally, emotionally, physically and spiritually in order for the relationship to flourish. The Dominant might hold the power in their hands but only as long as they keep within the boundaries that the Sub sets. This relationship is not an abusive one, the hurt is consensual with the Dom making sure the Sub is okay with the use of belts or whips or whatever other instruments they employ before letting loose with them.

They would probably begin slowly, in order for both parties to get comfortable and ensure that it's not just the idea of pain that is appealing but the application as well. Starting small can look like grabbing hold of the hair and making the other party perform oral sex on the Dom. In addition to sexual gratification, the Dom may also want to test the Sub's level of obedience. The Sub might be blindfolded during the exercise and the Dom might use a whip or a belt on them. The Dom might apply the belt hard enough to leave welts but rarely scars unless the Sub is up for that, just as long as the Sub is turned on by these activities and very often, they are. They love it. It might make them feel overwhelmed with emotion afterwards in the beginning. The feeling of having no control and loving it might be very new to them. The intensity of feelings unleashed might cause the new Sub to pull away for a while. The turn on for the sex Submissive is the surrender. They are willing to venture into areas many people wouldn't or couldn't. It is not a sign of weakness as many Subs are alphas in their normal lives – this might even be the reason why they feel the need to surrender in bed.

Because BDSM is about so much more than the physical sex act, a Dom can still apply his duties from far away. It is a matter of psychological control. The Sub will let the Dom know that they are about to do something; go for a run, cook, masturbate and the Dom can give permission or withhold it. The Dom can watch as the Sub masturbates until they are close to completion and then order them to stop. If the Sub goes against these agreed upon parameters, the Dom can punish them by not speaking to them for days on end or other ways that make them feel the sting of rejection.

There is always a safe word which is used to halt proceedings if the Sub can't take anymore. For example the Dom can make the Sub sit on their knees while the Dom spanks them. The safe word can be employed if the spanking becomes too much or they are unable to sustain their position on their knees. Many times, this safe word goes unused in spite of, or because of, the pain and misery of the position. This scenario emphasizes how important trust is in the d/s relationship even more than is usual in a normal, vanilla relationship. It is intoxicating for the Dom to be trusted so fully and for a Sub, to be able to surrender so fully is also intoxicating. The surrender doesn't come from a place of weakness. In fact, sex Submissives are sometimes willing to delve deep into places vanilla couples fear to tread. The physical pain is just one aspect of it. There is also surviving and enduring it which is a feat in anyone's book. If they can survive the pain, endure the suffering without demur, then what can't they do?

Being a sex Submissive might be a difficult thing to share with friends who might not understand. Many people in these relationships have chosen to hide it from those near and dear to them. Nobody wants to be judged. On the other hand, nobody wants to live in the closet forever. The emergence of Fifty Shades of Grey in popular literature has meant that people are sharing their baser fantasies and kinks more openly and this is great for the culture. On the other hand, representation matters. And Christian Grey is portrayed as a damaged or broken. This is an inaccurate portrayal of the average Dom and contributes to misunderstandings about the culture. Yes it's true that they may seem controlling when they tell the Sub what to wear to work or when to come, but it is all consensual.

In BDSM Subspace refers to the alternate reality which has its own properties, rules and texture in which the practice of BDSM takes place within a relationship. This Subspace can be present in the mind although the participants can alter their physical surroundings to better reflect their mental state. Physical space can consist of dungeons or private play rooms specifically designed to facilitate BDSM and get the participants in the mood and headspace to enjoy themselves to the maximum. It also allows them to strip away their everyday personas with their accompanying burdens, worries and responsibilities and really throw themselves into the roles they're playing.

Subspace means that specific psychological mentality in which the Sub is existing while in play with the Dom. In order to surrender themselves wholly to the Subspace, the Sub must completely trust the Dom so that they can give up complete control to their partner. In a way, being in the Subspace is similar to the practice of basic mindfulness. The similarities are the need to be present in the moment with your partner; this is a technique also used by athletes and entertainers when they are about to perform to get in the zone.

In the Subspace, all the Sub's feelings are intensified and their mind and emotions are immersed in the present moment. This space has no room for burdens or worries or responsibilities. They are free of the need to make decisions or think. All they have to do is obey.

Pain Submissives

Not every Submissive enjoys some form of pain but some do. They consider their bodies not only unique and special and also their responsibility to keep it safe, but also an instrument for their Dominant's enjoyment. The level of pain enjoyed by different Submissives vary from mild to extreme. The relationship they have with pain is different from that of vanilla people because they derive satisfaction and enjoyment from certain types of pain. These types of Submissives could be labeled as masochists since they derive sexual and emotional satisfaction from pain. Not only are they emotionally gratified when the Dominant inflicts pain on them to garner obedience or ensure dedication but they also require for pain to be present for them to be sexually gratified in some forms of sexual pleasure.

There is a difference between the debilitating pain of illness and that deliberately inflicted to a pain Submissive. Many pain Submissives simultaneously suffer from chronic pain and this changes the relationship they have with their bodies as masochists. This type of pain is not part of the kink and is known as undesirable pain and it is an issue that is dealt with within the culture.

There are different labels given to pain that is pleasurable vis-a-vis that which is undesirable. Subs often refer to these two types of pain as hurt vs. harm. When dealing with chronic pain, this distinction is even more important. Even outside of the BDSM world, these distinctions do exist. There is pain that is associated with wellness and getting better that does not drain the individual in a physical and emotional way whereas bad pain is defined as being debilitating to both body and spirit.

Pain Submissives take a great deal of pride in being able to hold up in the face of heavy impact play. They are proud of the bruises they get when they are caned and would be happy to show off the split open skin, purple bruises and welts. When they are unable to endure even a simple whipping it makes them feel like a failure, they are ashamed of their inability to take it. They feel like they have failed as a Submissive if they cannot endure the pain.

This is an internal reaction, having nothing to do with the Dominant. It is a personal failure.

This reaction is quite common among masochists if they have to invoke the safe word because of inability to endure pain. This is especially so if they were previously able to endure that level of pain in play.

When that happens, it is essential that a new play plan is formulated in which the pain Submissive can participate and feel good about it, without having to invoke the safe word. This might involve such things as bondage or sensation play.

The difference in pain thresholds among masochists might be explained by endorphin levels. Most people, especially those in the BDSM lifestyle, have heard of endorphins although they might not understand how they work or what the 'endorphin high' is.

This high comes about when the body pumps a number of morphine-like chemicals into the brain. These chemicals lower the body's sensitivity to pain thus raising its pain threshold. The body releases endorphins in measured loads and it is possible to manipulate one's body into releasing an endorphin pack. The body then takes about ten minutes to put together another pack if there is proper stimulation to do so. This stimulation might consist of light paddling, light caning, sensation play or flogging. The intensity of the Subsequent stimulation does not have to match that which caused the initial endorphin release. Once this groundwork has been set, it might take only five minutes to achieve climax which again triggers release of more endorphins. This cycle is dependent upon the Submissive's current threshold of pain, and how it is calculated to push them over the new edge.

This means that when the d/s couple begins the scene, the amount of endorphins in the Submissive is zero. This also means that infliction of any type of pain from a pinch to a light slap will garner a pained reaction. This causes emergency reserves of endorphins to be released in the case of the mildest pain which then builds to a gentle climax. This causes a jump in the threshold of pain. This makes it easier for the Sub to tolerate higher levels of pain with less reaction. This new level of pain tolerance is known as level one. The state of consciousness is not changed but the amount of pain that can be tolerated is higher.

At this point, the Dom spends the next ten minutes in play that causes fairly light but steady stimulation in order to encourage the body to assemble the next pack of endorphins. This might consist of whipping, flogging or paddling which doesn't demand a lot of energy exertion from the Dom.

After the next ten minutes have expired, the Dom will seek to increase the intensity of sensation for the next five minutes in order to drive the body to climax. This is followed by rapid fire ten to fifteen seconds of intense stimulation just creeping past the point of pain endurance for the Sub thus causing a fresh ejection of endorphin into the bloodstream. This takes the Sub to level two, without changing their state of consciousness in any noticeable manner except for panting and other signs of exertion. However, the pain threshold rises significantly and obviously. More light stimulation for the next ten minutes leads to another load generation, this time significantly under the new threshold of pain and kept there by the occasional heavy thwack of a whip or cane, about one minute apart. This keeps adrenalin building at minimal levels.

After this, the Dom can take a break and relax for ten minutes. Then it's back to slowly building up that intensity for five minutes, well above the previous threshold. The Sub has a very high pain threshold by now and is able to take more pain than is usual for what would normally be considered crisis level. This triggers the next release of endorphin which culminates in ten seconds to a minute of extreme effort to push the body to release the load.

Having now entered level three, the hormonal levels in the Sub's body has them a little dizzy and looking drugged. The Sub's eyelids might fall closed and they will be very relaxed, and less inhibited, probably making noises to indicate their new level of euphoria such as moans and groans.

This cycle is repeated again only with a more intensified climax at the end of it that releases the next load of endorphins and ups the ante to level four head space. In this Subspace, the state of consciousness is changed to a very loose, drugged feel, relaxed, compliant Submissive offset by the large amounts of adrenaline that have also been produced by the massive climax experienced at the end of level three. The Submissive's state at this time can be said to be relaxed yet hypersensitive. They are still able to communicate and react to stimuli. The lightest tap with a cane or whip would produce a hyper reaction in form of twitches and jerking around. This means that when they are indulging in ten minute light stimulation the Sub's response is more vocal, more intense, more uninhibited. The Dom is required to do very little at this time to stimulate even more reaction. The threshold of pain is very high although reaction time increases due to the presence of adrenalin. If the Dom should choose to hit a bit harder occasionally, this sensation is definitely welcome and the Submissive may ask for more.

If sexual play is part of the process, this should take place somewhere around level three. The higher the levels go, the less able the Submissive is to concentrate on what's going on. The result might be a very passionate encounter free of inhibitions or inability to perform. There is no way to predict which way it will go.

When endorphins are replenished during the Subsequent ten minute period, it is important for the Dom to pay attention to the limits reached on previous levels as the five minute build up starts again. The purpose here is to take the Sub to a place of in extremis as their pain threshold is at its highest and, while having the Sub simultaneously out of it, and they may not be able to say the safe word. The Sub might not even be in a state to think to use the safe word. It is therefore necessary for the Dom to exercise sensitivity and finesse as they pay attention to their Sub's every reaction. This session might last ten to thirty seconds and culminate in a final blast of endorphins that elevates the Sub to the fifth level which is a state of extreme docility, ecstasy and compliance with anything the Dom does.

Usually, unless the Sub indicates otherwise, this is the point at which aftercare takes place where the Sub will be covered in a blanket and taken care of by the Dom.

Domination

So, we've looked at things from the perspective of being a submissive. But what is it like from the other side: being the dominator? Just like the submissive, the dominator can take many different forms. It involves committing completely to one's partner and earning their trust. The partnership between S&D is extremely intimate and the submissive could feel emotionally and physically vulnerable. But far from what some people believe, the S&D relationship is not a punitive, abusive one but one of love at its deepest level. The dominator may be answering the needs of the submissive, which stem from a deep-seated psychological concept planted imperceptibly many years before they met. By the very fact that the submissive trusts his or her partner with their innermost personal fantasies, which they may not have shared with anyone else, requires an intimacy born out of love and mutual respect or at least it should.

Typically, the inclination to be a submissive originates from a desire to please another person at a very profound level and this involves submitting to them and relinquishing any control. It is about giving away the right to make your own decisions. This can permeate into all areas of your life or in specific ones only. Equally, to be a dominator requires a desire to be in control of another person and to have them hand over their personal power to you. It can be either gender who takes on this role, but statistically, it is currently the male role even though this is constantly changing as more women realize the benefits of being the dominator. It also involves different kinds of domination and might cut across just one or expand to all areas of a couple's lives, as outlined below. Try and rid your mind of the sub suffering unimaginable pain, which will never stop despite how they beg. True S&D is a considered practice that has been discussed and measured by both members of the couple. It is a negotiation. And that is usually negotiation between people who love each other deeply and would never knowingly hurt one another, either physically or emotionally.

Financial Domination

This is also called "findom." One partner has complete control over the finances. So perhaps they don't have a joint bank account and only one person has control of the account. If they both work, then it goes into the same account and the one who is not in control receives an allowance. They can be made to present all receipts for expenditure to the other person. One person can also have power of attorney over the other so that they are allowed to sign anything their partner would be. All property can be assigned to one person too. This regime demands enormous trust because of course should the relationship break up this would cause hugely complicated problems for the party who has relinquished all their rights to the other. Commit to this with caution.

Nevertheless, as extreme as this might sound, it does have benefits. If only one person is in control, it centralizes financial organization and ensures there is no duplication of bills being paid or that something is being overlooked. Financial domination can be extremely empowering for the person in control and also act as a stress reliever for the person on an allowance.

Domestic Dominance

Traditionally, of course, it has always been the women who has stayed at home and looked after the household but, as roles in the work arena change, so too does the person who takes charge of the domestic chores. If both parties are working, then it might be preferable that chores can be shared out between the couple but this equality is not always fully adopted, and this might be by design. Alternatively, men are more often becoming househusbands and assuming total control. This is most often when the woman in the partnership earns significantly more than her partner, but it might also be a considered decision. One person might be much better at cooking, cleaning and all things domestic but alternatively someone can be taught to improve at any task given the right incentive which may or may not be sex related.

Childcare

Women are more likely than not to have the larger responsibility for the raising of the children of the family. Men can often fail to appreciate how stressful this sometimes is, negotiating peak time traffic and having loud demands being met on them by children who insist on acting their age. However, both the father and the children can benefit by the deeper impact of a father who introduces a different and possibly more masculine dynamic into their lives and shapes their development in a far different way to the mother.   It is conceivable that this will change over time as roles within society change too and influence family relationships and dynamics further.

The domina or dominator feels the need for control of another person for a variety of reasons. It may be that the relationship is the only area of their lives where they have this opportunity. It does not necessarily stem from a need to be cruel or abuse another person and, in fact, it is probably quite the reverse. The dominator trusts the other person sufficiently to invest their trust and deepest confidences to them. It's a comfort to let someone else take control and provide release from everyday stresses and pressures. This used to be more accurate for the men in our society because they were the ones who were expected to be the strong alpha males who protected their weaker sex women.

For centuries, it has been the man who has been portrayed – probably quite accurately – as the one who was in charge: of the household; of the money and thus of the sex life he wanted. His financial dominance controlled everything else because his wife was obviously dependent upon him to maintain her own and possibly the couple's children's maintenance. His wife complied with his wishes because if she didn't there would be nowhere else for her to live, so she didn't seem to have much choice. But in romantic novels and even modern chic flicks, the man can still be seen to be sweeping the damsel in distress off her feet or charming the pants off her at least. (Think as recently as Brigit Jones when women's equality had to be mixed with humor and romance to be credible). Normally, the language in chick flick romance is flowery and while the little lady beats the chest of the man protesting how much she doesn't want him to kiss her, he pulls her tightly to him, ignoring her pleas. She swoons and melts into his embrace, enjoying having his tongue pushed down her throat, no doubt as a prelude to a hot night of steamy sex when she is subjected to anything he might fancy at the time and, of course, which she has no power to resist. As if.

How many women have enjoyed this fantasy – on a theme – as they lay in bed with their partners during another deadly boring interlude that had come to be accepted as an acceptable sex life between them? For a woman who does not feel it taboo to be desiring an alternative, striking out and asking for more should add an extra dimension for both partners in the relationship. Living out this fantasy for women allows them to kick a vanilla society, which has expected them to be pure and adorable, in the teeth. They want dirty sex that allows them to be their partner's slave and be totally controlled by him and told what to do. Sleazy is appealing. They actually want to be treated as a sex object, no matter how much they might protest otherwise. (Take me, take me, no matter how much I protest but remember the safe word too). For women, sex is a cerebral activity and more of it happens in that part of the body than anywhere else. Perhaps it helps feeling guilty because this sort of sex is still taboo to a certain extent and they want to revel in the naughtiness of it all. They want to be owned by a man, totally possessed and dominated.

Some examples of a way a dominator might treat his partner might be that he ties her to the bed, totally naked, with her legs splayed. He then goes out on an errand and leaves her there. He might tell someone to pop in to get something that he borrowed from them and it's in the bedroom but he could make up some excuse why it is essential that they should go and get it now. When they get to the bedroom, they see his partner splayed out on the bed. She might even be blindfold so doesn't know who is there looking at her. But she is totally helpless. When he gets back, she asks him why he came into the room earlier and then left her there again, and he tells her that it was one of the neighbors but he won't say which one. If they wanted to take this further, he could have told the neighbor to help himself to whatever he fancied and it was up to the neighbor if he jumped on her and took her partner at his word. This would be incredibly erotic for both partners, especially if the male was into cuckolding.

Another fantasy might be that the woman is either dressed up erotically or that she is totally naked. Her partner puts a dog collar around her neck and leads her around the house on it. She has to stay on all fours to drink and eat and she also has to suck his cock on demand. She has to rest in a dog basket and when he calls her over he takes her from behind. If the couple is into voyeurism, then they could invite others and have a party.

Women often enjoy being spanked too and can find it especially pleasurable to go over their partner's knee for a spanking. The man should pull down the woman's panties and maybe finger her a little. Just as she is beginning to enjoy it and starts to moan, he will spank her and tell her to be silent. When he has spanked her a few times, he will begin spanking her again until she can hardly stand it anymore. He should leave her panties around her thighs or knees and then tell her to stand up and remove her top and put one of her breasts into his mouth because he wants to suck it. When he is good and ready he can fuck her to his cock's content.

Although the woman has historically been in charge of the housework, she could become his slave for the weekend for instance – or longer if they wish – domestically and sexually. This might involve doing the vacuuming in nothing but stockings and high heels and an apron. If she doesn't do a good enough job to please him, she has to get down on all fours and suck his dick. He could also spank her as well. She is not allowed any sex herself because she is only there to please him and has not earned any treats. She can also use her hands to masturbate him. He might also insist that she has sex with another woman because that has always been one of his fantasies or with someone he brings home from the bar. She agrees because she knows that he is her master and she must obey him or she will be punished.

For a man, being the dominator confirms his masculinity. In society at large, he may otherwise feel emasculated to a degree but in his own home, and with the partner he loves, he is treated as king, he who must be obeyed. For a partner to be able to put his wife over his knee and spank her is highly satisfying for him. He makes her agree that he is boss in his own house and that she must submit to his desires at any time he wishes. Imagine having sex on demand anytime he wishes, or having his cock sucked at any time when within other couples where the man is not dominant, she may refuse to do it when he wants or at all. He would be able to touch her in any part of her body whenever he chooses and she must submit. It also works for the female submissive though because she is a little girl again, free of conscious thoughts that prevail and spoil her fun. She has to relinquish all power to her husband, an action which is not too incredible and not too far removed from truth of not that long ago.

When a man wants to take the submissive role, it is normally because he wants to escape the stresses of his life. He might have a high powered role. Many politicians or empire magnets have sexual proclivities along this vein. They take great pleasure living out the fantasy of having no will of their own and submitting completely to another person, albeit someone that they might share a deep and lasting bond and relationship with. It is highly sexual to have a confident, sassy lady in charge of their bodies, telling them what to do. Also, they might still associate the pain that a domina doles out to them with being chastised by the most dominant female in their childhood or adolescence when their sexuality was just awakening: their mother.

It is a relief for them to be able to hand over responsibility for being in charge of sex. It can also take the hard work out of things if he receives instruction about what the woman wants to happen or if she rides him on top instead of him having to maneuver into acrobatic positions to perform. More and more men enjoy becoming the sexual slaves of their partners. It is a relief to be able to disclose secrets they may have hidden all their lives and share their guilty secrets and have them made into reality. It might be the man who persuades his woman to dominate him, or it could even be the other way around these days as man's role in society is up for constant review and change.

When a man truly loves his partner he wants to please her, just as he did his mother. If a woman is clever, she will know how to exploit this so that they both benefit from it hugely. Why shouldn't a man romance his lady? And why shouldn't the lady accept it with good grace? There is nothing wrong with romance and domination could be just that: romance. Acting like a gentleman is an art long forgotten by many men and part of the reason could be because of women's rejection of it in their endless struggle to achieve emancipation. Equally, male submission can develop into the raunchiest sex that either of the couple has ever experienced but this should always be by negotiation and agreement.

If the man is the submissive, then it takes a strong and confident woman to be the domina. She is happy in her own skin and not afraid to ask for what she wants. She may tantalize the man by dressing up in leather or some other material he might have a fetish about. She can

55

control his orgasms, use cock and ball torture, chain him up, whip him, spank him, deny him sex. It's an endless list and always up for discussion and agreement.

Quite often the man might have carried fantasies of being dominated in his head for years but never had the confidence to ask his partner to cooperate. When he does find a partner he can truly trust, this is quite likely to be the time that he starts to live out those long-held fantasies. He may have been raised in a religious or strict home. Perhaps his mother thought the human body should never be seen and used only for procreation. She might even have reprimanded him for touching his own genitals. It is no wonder then that he feels that sex is somehow dirty and carries lots of sexual baggage around, lots of it in knots in his head that his mother helped to tie from a very early age. It may take lots of discussion and understanding from a partner to unravel this confusion and to help him live a satisfying and fulfilling sex life, one where he does not feel like a freak or pervert.

Different scenarios, which are set out are suggestions only and should be adapted to your own requirements, but might be as follows.

Your partner insists that you run her a bath with bubbles or oil. She also requires you to be naked. You should get her a glass of wine and light a lot of candles around the bath. This scenario is more along the lines of romance. When she has finished, you have to shave her pubes, paint her nails and then massage her body with oil. You must then perform any sexual act on her that she demands. It is up to her whether or not she allows you any sexual gratification.

Another suggestion might be when she tells you to strip off and ties you face down to a table. She paddles your ass until you beg her to stop and then to punish you she puts on a strap-on dildo and makes you suck it before fucking you with it until you scream out for her to stop.

If she wants a domestic slave, one which all women should take advantage of, you must strip off and only wear an apron. She gives you jobs around the house and tells you if you do them well you will be allowed to lick out her pussy and if you're really good it might be more too. However, if you do not do a good job and she is not satisfied with your work, she will bend you over and whip your ass. If you have finished a particular job in time, you will be allowed a ten-minute break and allowed to eat lunch. Lunch, however, will be eaten from a dish on the floor because you are not worthy to sit at the table with her. If she is not happy with you, she will also spit on you and you will have to lick her toes.

As already stated above, these are only suggestions. No doubt you both have your own ideas or you might have ideas on how you can adapt the above. Either way, remember you are doing this to have fun. Get rid of the guilt, loosen up and get stuck in. However, be warned: once you have started to have this type of sex with abandon it can be so good that it gets addictive and you may never want to return to a bland vanilla sex life again. In fact, it is likely to just keep on getting dirtier as you experiment to find something new to excite you more.

Boundaries

Because BDSM can be out there and can get very physical, it is important to draw up guidelines between you for what is and is not acceptable. This might also apply to emotional boundaries too. Quite often, you can find that treading unknown territory can touch nerve ends and bring up painful things from the past, which you thought you'd dealt with or at least subdued. It's not a bad thing to bring these memories back out of the box where you thought they'd remain forever. Discussing hurtful things that might well have driven your sexual motivations is liberating and empowering, freeing you up to a more enjoyable sex life and a much deeper understanding with your partner. How much more can be divulged than secrets that you may never have told anyone else? You are revealing your innermost thoughts as well as surrendering your body to what may be punishing treatments and trusting that other person with everything you have.

You both need to sit down and discuss at length a prescription which you can both agree to. Why do you have negative feelings? When did you first realize that you wanted to participate in this kind of sex? Why do you think it is taboo? Hopefully, discussions should run smoothly. Listen to each other with an open mind and be non-judgmental. Perhaps it would be helpful to draw up a contract agreeing on what is acceptable and what is not. This might include:

Health and Safety

This is first because it is probably the most important one. BDSM is a very physical way of having sex, sometimes including using instruments or appliances with a varying degree of risk. If you are using these, be sure you know how they operate. If in doubt at all, then research fully how that particular item should be used. The last thing you want to do is end up causing permanent physical – or emotional – damage. If you are using a paddle, whip or belt, for instance, you should experiment with the amount of pain you can inflict. Everyone has different pain thresholds and what you think you can withstand might be totally different from your partner's. Women often say that if they can survive childbirth for instance, then they can get through anything. However, some women suffer horrendous labor that goes on for days while others shed babies like peas. Pain tolerance is totally unique.

Safe Word

To help you regulate how much pain either partner can tolerate, having a safe word is a good idea. Decide on something between you that is a word that you would not normally use in the normal course of conversation: boomerang, flipper, anchor. But most definitely do not make it stop. Even used as STOP is not a good idea, as this could be used in times of erotic, exotic sex when the dominator thinks his partner is simply saying as part of the game. Use this only when the pain really is too much to bear because if it used too frequently it becomes meaningless and perhaps this is not the right type of sex for you??

Child Protection

Never participate in BDSM when the children are at home. Either get someone to babysit in your home and you go away for the night, or get the babysitters to take the kids to their own home. If you are using any equipment, magazines, books, movies then please lock them away in a very safe place. Don't leave the key where the children can get at it. Who wouldn't like to investigate a locked box?

Privacy

Sometimes involving someone else can be part of the game. You might be able to stay under the radar and be anonymous in a big metropolitan district. But in a small community finding out that you and your partner practice BDSM could soon earn you the name of the local perverts. Your job is not to educate those people who are still locked in the cell of vanilla sex and who are they to judge you anyway? Don't give them any ammunition. Who knows what might get back to your boss or your children's schoolmates? Keep your own counsel.

Deprivation of breath

It wouldn't be advisable to use this for sexual stimulation because it can be highly dangerous. When people do use it, they do it by using plastic bags over the head or choking. This deprives the brain of much needed oxygen and creates a feeling of giddiness, lightheadedness and a high which is much like that given by cocaine. It can be highly addictive but it can also be fatal. Don't go there.

Golden Showers

Many enjoy their partners to urinating on them. They want to be degraded and feel this is an excellent way of fulfilling that wish. Some drink it and while it is not harmful in small quantities it would not be a good idea to drink it regularly or in large amounts.

Human Toilet Paper

This is a definite no-no. While some may find this pleasurable it is an extremely dangerous activity and could cause serious health problems ranging from diarrhea to liver problems.

Disability

If one of you is disabled or has health problems, you can still engage in BDSM but you must adopt the necessary actions for the disability or illness. For instance, for someone with a heart complaint, physical chastisement or vigorous sex could kill them. So you should go forward very gently and slowly, doing research when needed.

Mental Health

As mentioned earlier, engaging in new forms of sexual practice can easily bring up old issues that you may have thought were put to bed and laid to rest. Methods covered by BDSM can trigger something in the brain, which can in turn release old and painful memories. If this is the case in your partnership, then either discuss things at length with your partner or seek counseling from a qualified practitioner. This is not to suggest that you are outside of the norms. We are all carrying baggage. Perhaps the more daring you become and push the boundaries by sexual experimentation the more you release yourself, not just sexually but holistically. Rest assured that we all have our hang-ups. Our brains are so complex that we kick and protest against thoughts we have been so well trained to believe are perverse or perverted. How much effort does it take to shake those harmful restrictions and move forward into the life we deserve? With the help of a loving partner, it becomes so much easier to adopt the life we have been seeking and denied.

Impact Play

This is hitting your partner either with the palm of your hand or an instrument such as a paddle or whip. Check out where the main organs in the body are and avoid them so you do not damage them. The best part to hit someone is either the fleshy part of the ass or just underneath when the cheek joins the top of the leg and which can be quite erotic.

Cuckolding

Is one or both of you interested in cuckolding? It can be a dangerous thing to do to involve someone else in your sex lives so you must be absolutely sure that this is what you want to do. Obviously, it could be perceived as cheating even if the partner is in the loop and bring feelings of extreme jealousy to the fore. Proceed with caution. Saying this, it can be an incredibly erotic practice, but you should be sure you are not playing with fire.

Alcohol and Drugs

It might be a bad idea to alter or dull your senses when you are experimenting with corporal punishment or sex equipment and toys. A dulled sense of pain tolerance could be a detriment to measuring the strength of pain administered. A glass of wine or two might be a good idea to help you relax and overcome inhibitions but a bottle or two or a line of cocaine should be avoided. Who needs highs from substances when your endorphins should be shooting through the roof with pleasure from the sex session you're having? Imbibing more than you should, might lead to you forgetting the whole experience. You should be remembering every toe tingling second of your erotic adventures.

Going Public

Do you and your partner want others to know? Are you sick of hiding who you really are and you are so comfortable with your role that you feel you have nothing to hide and don't care who knows, then go for it. However, you must both be in complete agreement and be sure that it will not jeopardize the job prospects of either of you or have a negative impact on someone you love or who loves you such as a child or your own elderly mother, who might struggle to come to terms with something she could never have conceived actually existed. Exhibitionism might be part of your sexual inclinations and a good way of doing this is by going to clubs that cater specifically for those practicing BDSM. At the very least, it's a good night out and you should dress up in the part to go. Otherwise, it will be you who stands out from the crowd when you get there and take off your coat. You are likely to meet many larger than life, colorful people who are likely to push your life into a different arena. You do not have to necessarily join in with the activities and can go just to meet people or to get some new ideas to do in the privacy of your own home. Many of these clubs have playrooms that include bondage equipment and there might be a room where a mass of people enjoy communal sex. But before you do decide to go to one of these clubs, you must both be very clear about the level of participation you want to have. Perhaps the first visit could be a recce for you to see the lie of the land before agreeing to anything. When you have a clearer idea you can always go back and join in, even if it's only gradually. At the very least, it will enable you to meet others who enjoy the same sort of things that you and your partner do and for you both to develop a group identity that is probably new to you.

Absolutely No Go Areas

Hopefully, the majority has been instilled with a very effective moral compass who would never agree to do anything that might hurt others. This absolutely includes rape or murder, of course.

It also includes emotional blackmail. If your partner says that they do not wish to participate in a particular activity, never try and force them to do so or use emotional blackmail to make them feel bad and do something they really are averse to doing. If you both agree what is reasonably acceptable and then one partner ignores this rule and oversteps the mark, this is abuse in its cruelest of forms: sexual, emotional, physical, and you are abusing the power in the relationship that your partner has agreed to imbue you with. Ignore this at our peril because if you betray the agreement, you have only yourself to blame if your partnership disintegrates. Absolutely, never ever abuse anyone who is emotionally vulnerable or having a low point in their lives. Never EVER prey on someone who is not legally of age and this should encompass people who might have special needs. If you cross this line, you are guilty of abuse both physically and emotionally. In no one's perception, can this be acceptable. In fact, if you do feel as if you want to take advantage of someone who is underage or mentally vulnerable, this is outside of the boundaries of what is acceptable. Indeed, it is illegal and you could be quite rightfully legally prosecuted. If you have feelings like this, you should most definitely seek professional help for your mental health. Equally, this applies if you are physically cruel or particularly aggressive towards your partner. If they are not in agreement, then your behavior is not normal. If you are in any doubt whatsoever, and our partner is expressing negative sentiments, seek help immediately.

Public Humiliation between Female Friends

This might be verbal abuse in front of others and is covered much more thoroughly in a later part and in much more absolute detail. The woman might joke among her friends while her partner is there that she had him working all night trying to satisfy her because he just could not get it right. She might make him the butt of jokes and make her friends laugh at his expense. This should only be done with an agreement because without it, it could be perceived as a total betrayal of trust. On the other hand, if the partner gets turned on with it, all systems are go. The female could also make her partner dance in front of her female friends as a form of entertainment. She then instructs him to go to bed, perhaps after spanking him in front of her friends, who all applaud when he shouts out and begs for mercy.

Drawing up an Agreement

A list does not have to be elaborate and could contain a simple list of bullet points. No doubt you have already had a lot of discussions about what turns you on and what you could not tolerate by any stretch of the imagination so it should be a very simple exercise. Maybe the left side says what is acceptable and the right side says what is not. This should be done on a regular basis; in fact, it might be a good idea to quickly skim through it before any session because what was quite acceptable one day may be totally reversed the next. Another reason why it does not have to be minutely detailed is that there has always got to be some element of spontaneity. To know exactly what is coming every time might be heading back along the path to vanilla sex. Use common sense and if in doubt your partner always has the safe word. Never abuse that or disregard it.

These are just the obvious ones and no doubt you could add more of your own. If so, add them to your agreement, which you should both sign and date every time you adjust it at all. If you're the submissive partner, don't let your partner persuade you that you should take more pain than you feel comfortable with because it is part of the practice. This is abuse. Never be afraid to stand up and say that you do not agree with it. Your sexual experience is being expanded because you want it that way. This fantastic journey is a revelation for both parties and whichever role they adopt, both should benefit equally and share a much deeper bond than they knew previously.

CHAPTER THREE
Subcultures

The Slave

This form of Submission has the Submissive surrendering every aspect of their will to their master. It is a more extreme and consuming type of Submission where the Sub is not the one who decides what their boundaries are, but have those limits set for them by their Dom or master/mistress. They behave as if their Dom owns them and in many cases, wear collars to indicate their 'owned' status.

Many people dispute the assertion that a slave is a Submissive. This is because their lifestyle is generally more extreme than the Submissive's life by normal standards. While the Submissive has a broad spectrum of spaces in which to fit, there are some commonalities. On one side of the spectrum is being a Sub only within the bedroom walls on the other side, it may extend to every aspect of your life. The core of being a Submissive is the distinct choice one makes to Submit and there being a safe word which is really the choice of saying 'no' to some aspect of play should they wish to. The Submissive is the one who chooses which aspects of their lives are going to be ceded to the Dominant and that power exchange is voluntary.

Therefore, the question arises, how can consensual slavery be considered part of the Submissive culture? The whole premise behind being a slave is commitment to obedience. They are not expected to ask questions or to have self-chosen boundaries. They do as they are told regardless of the extremity or their own thoughts on the Subject. When the Dominant gives them an order, they are expected to obey it regardless of how they may feel about it. The slave surrenders total control of their selves to the Dominant as far as is humanly possible.

Both slaves and Submissives are variously described as property of their masters. In the former case however, they are literally considered to be owned by their masters as a matter of course and mutual consent. The slave commits to obey the Dom's every command. To break this deal by saying no means the end of the relationship.

It is therefore safe to say that a slave cannot be perceived as a higher form of Submissive. This hierarchy does not exist. The difference could be said to be the mindset of these two groups. The Submissive on one hand has a need to be told what to do whereas the slave needs to do what they are told. This is of course an oversimplification but for the purposes of illustration, would serve very well. The first part of the quote implies that Submissives require to be given guidelines or direction from the Dom as to how they should behave. Thus the concept is of training of the Sub by the Dom to fulfill their desires. This is also fits in with the concepts of reward and punishment that define these relationships. The Sub's mission is not necessarily to be obedient, but it is to please the Dom. Some Submissives wish to have the Dom make them obey by being bratty and that is also part of Sub culture.

Slaves, on the other hand, are hard wired to obey their Dom. That is the mantra under which they live. They are not necessarily trained to be so and are not rewarded for obeying. The film, Fifty Shades of Grey illustrates the Sub vs. slave debate by depicting the protagonist, Christian Grey, as wanting a 'contract slave.' The heroine, Anastasia, was however closer to a Submissive than a slave and a lesson for all Doms is that they should know their Subject very well.

Pet

The types of animals that pet play Submissives usually pretend to be include puppies, kittens or ponies. Pet play is enhanced by the use of costumes and accessories such as cages, collars and tails. There is a question as to what the Submissive gets out of pet play. Some might enjoy being dehumanized or the exhibitionism that goes along with pet play. Others enjoy surrendering their mental faculties and letting their owner pet and stroke them as if they were pets. This is, however, no relation to bestiality.

Of all the BDSM Subcultures, pet play is one of the least known and yet many of its adherents consider it one of the most fun part of being a Sub. Pet play reinforces the relationship between Dom and Sub in terms of being the owner vs. being owned. For ordinary pets, their survival completely depends on their human owners; whether or not they remember to feed them, vaccinate, provide somewhere for them to bed down or give them toys. This scenario is also true for a full time d/s relationship. In case of slavery, the slave eats after the master has eaten. They sleep where they are told and wear whatever the owner wants. Whatever rules the owner decides on must be followed to the letter. Thus for many Subs, being a pet to their Dom reinforces the relationship that they have with each other.

But how does a Sub choose which animal to be?

There are three typical ways that a Sub chooses a pet to become. The first one is instinctive, going for the animal with which they most identify. Loyal playful Subs might choose a puppy as their chosen pet to be while those that enjoy prancing about and lots of training might choose to be a pony.

The second way that a type of pet is chosen is for the Dominant to decide for the Submissive what they are going to be. The Dominant chooses the pet they prefer to deal with and then train the Sub into being that animal. For example a farmer Dom who enjoys milking might make his Sub a cow.

The third way that a pet to play is chosen might be to simply switch from animal to animal if they do not wish to commit to pet play as a long term thing. If it's all an experiment they will not necessarily choose just one animal.

How does pet play enhance the d/s relationship?

Many couples might choose pet play because of the dependency and humiliation. The Sub is restricted in how much they can vocalize their wants and needs, as well as how they move, eat, etc. thus they are much more dependent on the relationship that they have with their Dom to fulfill their needs. Humiliation comes in when a pet is not allowed to sit on the furniture or is forced to relieve themselves in a litter box rather than use the toilet.

Pet play can be used as a de-stressor when the Sub comes home from dealing with the daily challenges of life. They shed their human persona and mindlessly chase balls of twine or play with cat toys and get treats. Thus they escape from their minds and live only in their bodies, surrendering all decisions to the Dom.

Pet play might also help to center the Submissive as an instrument of the Dom's pleasure. Removing their humanity from them automatically puts them on a lower scale than their human Dom and this can help them adjust their mindset to letting the Dom be the decision maker in the relationship. It can also be used as a punishment for misbehavior. The recalcitrant Submissive might literally be placed in the doghouse and made to act like a dog as punishment.

Couples engage in pet play by having the Submissive's movement restricted using bondage, stopping them from speaking except for animal related words like woof and meow. Or else they are restricted to child-like words such as 'potty' or 'daddy' or 'up.'

While they are in pet mode, they might undergo 'house training' such as walking on a leash or lead, pulling a cart or sitting up and begging. The Submissive is fed from a pet bowl and is expected to eat with just their mouths. They relieve themselves by going in a litter box or being 'let out' to do it outside. They play with toys, use puppy whining to beg for treats, are caged in pet houses and are not allowed any human privileges such as sitting on the couch.

However as one dives into the world of pet play, it is important to observe certain rules for their own safety. For example when pretending to be an animal, it is not safe to eat pet food on a regular basis. The human metabolism is much different from that of animals and so their nutritional needs vary. It is possible to pretend to eat animal foods by shaping human food into looking like animal feed. This can include baking biscuits in the shape of dog bones.

When carrying out training, it is important that the Dom knows what they are doing. Anything that comes with instructions must be studied carefully before use such as shock collars. If one is fitting a 'puppy' into a kennel they must make sure the space is not too cramped; this could cause both short and long term damage to the pet. A form of communication needs to be set up with the pet so that they can convey distress or be able to call a halt in case of physical, or emotional injury. This illustrates how alert the

Dom must be to the Sub's needs especially in this situation. They must be aware of the added responsibility placed upon themselves to make sure that the Sub is kept safe.

Pet play might have sexual elements or might be completely nonsexual depending on the desires of the couple in question.

Little

A little is a type of baby, might be male or female, in an adult body. The little is in search of a positive male role model who can protect them. They fall somewhere between Submissive and pet in that they look up to their master or daddy Dom as a father figure. They desire to be protected and handled gently and with care and nurtured in their vulnerability. Being a little is not associated with playing a specific age, it is more about the nurturing, protective and supportive daddy Dom.

The little has the same needs as a baby and projects innocence and inner vulnerability, appearing like a child behavior-wise. This is not done in pretense and it is not some form of age play. The little and their daddy Dom are not playing out an incestuous or pedophilic fantasy. The little is simply an adult with a childlike personality who seeks a partner who is emotionally mature and nurturing. Daddy Doms can be defined as Dominants with that emotional maturity and caring nature needed by the little. The difference between daddy Doms and masters is the manner in which they choose to take control. Daddy Doms are concerned with the personal growth, needs and goals rather than on the rules and limits of the d/s relationship. The daddy Dom encourages the Little to explore their inner selves, to play and savor that side of their personalities. They are patient, fun loving and love to laugh just as one would be with a child. They can, however, be just as sadistic as normal Doms, just like Littles can still have a masochistic side.

The job of the daddy Dom is to be in control of the little; this involves guiding her in the achievement of her goals, protecting and loving her and nurturing her spirit. They do still get to experience sexual pleasure with the little however. They enjoy being the daddy because that's part of who they are and the little satisfies their need to nurture and protect.

Sissy maid

The sissy maid is usually a feminized male who takes on Domestic rules usually carried out by females. They adopt behavior and mannerisms that make them effeminate and follow the Dominant's lead in carrying out certain tasks as ordered. This would include wearing plugs, altering their bodies through plastic surgery, being tied up and deposited in the corner for hours, servicing the master or mistress and their friends and anything else the Dominant might come up with.

Sissy training is usually done as part of the overall BDSM lifestyle. It covers both sexual and nonsexual activities like Domestic chores, application of makeup and other accessories, using an enema, anal penetration or performing blowjobs. In the case of the male sissy maid, the Dominant usually prefers it if they are completely effeminate which includes shaving all their bodily hair and dressing in femme clothes. In more extreme cases, the male can undergo cosmetic surgery or take hormone pills in order to look more feminine. Sissy maid training is part of this indoctrination where the sissy dresses as a maid.

The uniform is usually skimpy and sexy, meant to show off the sissy's assets. She keeps this outfit on as she performs various household tasks as well as sexual acts, all the while keeping their Submissive persona. The sissy maid lifestyle is perfected over time as trust grows between the Dominant and Submissive and they both understand what they need. The goal of being a sissy maid is to be continuously humiliated by the Dominant and to serve the Dominant in various humiliating female roles. This could include servicing the master or mistress in public as well as their friends. Being disrespected in social gatherings or being made to do punishments such as being tied up in a corner as the master carries on with his life.

Brat

The term brat as used in the Submissive culture is controversial as some think it's a bit of a misnomer. This is because the brat Submissive has a tendency to be contrary and act out counter to their Dom's expectations. According to a self-confessed brat, the reason that they do this is to ensure that the Dominant is bringing their A-game. If they are given instructions which contain loopholes or weak spots, they do not feel confident and secure. They don't feel safe with the Dominant. Therefore they give them a hard time in order to make sure that whatever instructions are given are airtight. The brat can be a challenge for some Dominants and some may not even want to deal with them. Others might enjoy Subjugating the brat Submissive by keeping them in line when they try to act sassy.

In addition to feeling safe when they know that the Dominant has thought of every loop hole and sealed every escape from a punishment or humiliation; the brat is also bitchy and enjoys the process of ragging on their Dominant. Other Submissives might look down upon them as not 'real' or genuine but the brat considers that they are an elevated form of Submissive who demand more from the Dominant. Not all Submissives are created equal and some brats do try to switch on occasion. However they are happiest with a Dominant that is alpha enough to keep them in line.

There are certain prerequisites to owning a brat in order for both Dominant and Submissive to be happy in the relationship. The first is patience which is an absolute must. The brat goes out of their way to be exasperating especially in the early days when they are still feeling each other out.

The Dom must be prepared for a lot of tension headaches and a rise in blood pressure, frustration and anger when the brat is in full tantrum mode. It is at this point that the Dom will learn full self-control and also how to control the brat. Failure to which the relationship will probably not survive.

Should they get through the tantrums unscathed or only slightly singed, hopefully they both have enough of a sense of humor to laugh about it afterwards, realizing that the tantrum is not about hurt or disrespect per se. It is fun for the brat and the right type of Dom and may be a source of a rueful smile in the future when they think back on it.

The Dom needs to have sufficient imagination in order to control the brat. The latter are intelligent beings and tend to be devious as well. The Dom must be able to match or exceed them in being ingenuous when meting out punishments or anticipating what shenanigans they are likely to try next. The Dom might become a little paranoid in this relationship.

Such shenanigans might include 'trying out' the crop or paddle on the Dom with the premise that the master or mistress should try out all toys on themselves first to make sure of their quality. The Dom should expect to be paddled by the brat Sub in their quest to 'ensure quality.' That is if they cannot think of a way to preempt or dissuade this behavior. For example the Dom might order for the Sub to carry the crop in their mouths while on their hands and knees, using very specific language without loopholes so that the Sub never has the crop in their hands.

The brat has several well-known tactics such as inciting the Dom. They almost cannot help themselves as they 'talk back' to the Dom, they taunt them with statements such as 'is that all you got?' or being snarky, sassy or sarcastic. They use pet names that are meant to slightly denigrate or make fun of. They might say 'Master/Mistress is always right' if the Dom says something non-complimentary about themselves. And then bring it up on several Subsequent occasions.

The brat will play pranks on the Dom like hiding sex toys or lacing shoes together when the Dom is sleeping. They might Substitute massage oil for food coloring but what the Dom has to remember is that it's all meant in fun. The brat is simply trying to bring fun into the play and that is where having the same sense of humor comes in handy. Otherwise the Dom will forever be reaching for their blood pressure pills and meting out punishments.

If the brat is silent, this is probably a symptom that they are up to no good. The Dom must be very attentive in order not to be caught in the brat's traps. They will use coyness, puppy dog eyes and other faux innocent ruses to lure their Doms into their traps and then claim innocence afterward like they have no clue what happened.

The importance of ensuring that there are no loopholes in the Dom's orders cannot be overstated. The Dom must use very specific language or else they might find themselves in sticky situations. Telling the Sub to 'go and make coffee,' without specifying what to do with it after might result in the Submissive making the coffee and not bringing the Dom a cup. If the Dom tells the Sub to behave but does not specify what kind of behavior, the Sub might take it as a license to behave badly. The Dom needs to watch out for when the brat starts a sentence with 'You said' because this usually means that they have found the loophole in their instructions.

These brat shenanigans usually provoke certain reactions from the Dom. The most obvious reaction is fury; the Dom might feel annoyed with the Sub for complicating things or with themselves for not being more vigilant. Probably both.

The brat might be angling for a good spanking with all their shenanigans and an attentive Dom will give it to them. Most brats are fans of spanking and therefore this punishment is also a reward. Other fun punishments include counting orgasms. If the brat misses one then they have to start again from one. Or they can indulge in play such as bondage or flogging.

Sometimes, the Dom really means it when they punish the brat because they went too far. This means that the Dom needs to communicate clearly to the brat that they are being punished and what for. This could be as simple as letting them know how disappointed the Dom is with them. This is cutting to the Sub if meant sincerely and will result in the brat bending over backwards to please the Dom in following days. They could also be given a time out where they kneel silently in the corner and face the wall. The aim is denial of time they could be spending with you.

The punishments could also take a sexual turn in terms of denial of orgasm. The Dom brings the Sub right up to the edge of climax and then pulls back. The brat feels frustrated and the aim is to match the level of frustration that they brought to the Dom with their antics. This punishment is only effective when the brat and Dom know each other very well in order to pull it off.

The Dom can also try to reason with the brat and give them good reasons to stop with the brattiness. Dominants are still humans and have their own triggers boundaries. Discussing with the brat on what those boundaries are could lead to mutual respect for both the Dom's and the brat's boundaries. Sharing histories means greater trust and better communication between them which enhances the relationship.

The Dom might also perfect a Look, which when leveled against the brat means that they need to back down now. If the look is effective, the brat will heed it and calm down. It is usually the first thing that a Dom will try when the brat is acting up.

When the brat gets too much, however, just stopping whatever activity you are doing might do the trick. It serves to focus their minds if the Dom just goes quiet and sits back, arms crossed. Addition of the Look to this activity might be effective in pulling the brat back from the brink. This is only possible if the brat respects the Dom and trusts them.

The finger snap is used by many Doms as a trigger to let the Sub know that they require their full attention. They are to stop whatever they are doing and focus on the Dom. The brat needs to be trained to respond automatically to the finger snap. This is done by indicating to the brat that the Dom wishes for something to be done. Like any other Submissive, the brat wants to make the Dom happy. With time and training, the finger snap will be an effective tool to focus the brat's attention immediately.

There are pet peeves that the brat might have which they want to use as one of their boundaries. If the Dom does not want a precedent set on setting hard limits on each and every pet peeve, they should not allow it to happen even once. Pet peeves might include things like tickling, where the brat might beg the Dom to stop.

PART TWO

Building a Great
Submissive Relationship

CHAPTER FOUR
Principles of a Healthy Relationship

The d/s or m/s relationship is based on a power dynamic that might last only when the two people are within sight and sound of each other or could be an ongoing thing. In order for this dynamic to work in a healthy way, certain principles must be put in place.

The first one is consent and a strong desire. Any relationship begins with consent but due to the power dynamic, this is especially so with d/s relationships. The

Submissive should be able to choose to participate because they want it, and every day, they continue to make the choice to stay. If trust is present then there is no need for shackles.

Some people are very persuasive and can convince someone to be in a Submissive relationship for a limited time, even if it's not really their thing. It is even possible to convince a susceptible person to live the lifestyle if one is convincing enough. However without consent and desire, the foundations of that relationship are extremely unstable at best and both participants are unlikely to derive any satisfaction from it.

When one gives consent, it might be assumed that this consent is forever but that is not the case. A long term couple might reach the point where it is not necessary to express that consent verbally because of the trust and symbiosis between them, however that does not mean it disappears. It simply becomes an intrinsic part of the relationship. This is because the two have established channels of verbal and nonverbal communication that transcend the need to articulate every thought. This is not always the case and it certainly takes a long time to reach this state of being. Everyone else just has to use their words.

It is important that the d/s couple distinguish between what is fantasy and what is reality. Role play takes place within the environment of d/s but if one is doing it 24/7 then there is more than that involved. Arousal and orgasm are integral parts of the d/s lifestyle but there are reasons beyond that that people commit to it full time. It is simply heightening the power dynamic of the relationship into everyday situations. Despite the fact that the power dynamic continues outside of the bedroom does not mean that the entire relationship is some sort of role play scenario. If an attempt is made to make the role play into an entire relationship what will happen is that instead of a couple in a relationship, you end up with a couple of characters who are not real. These characters cannot fulfill the needs of the holistic person because behind the character will be a person who has Subjugated themselves into playing a role. The Submissive might be able to act a role for a short period of time but if they do it 24/7 then that reduces the realness of the relationship.

So when being a full time Submissive regardless of what they are wearing, where they are or what they are doing means some adjustment to cater for outside stimuli. The Submissive might ramp up or reduce the visibility of their Submissive tendencies depending on whether they are in public, at work or at home, alone with their Dominant. They may not be able to maintain classic Submissive roles all the time.

The choice that the Submissive makes to live this lifestyle must be done from a place of strength. The motivation must come from a place of pure want and not because of a perceived dependence on the lifestyle in order to function. Dysfunction and Submissiveness is not the same thing. Should the Submissive discover that they have a dysfunction, they need to address it separately.

Thus the Submissive must be committed to work on their issues since the intensity of the power dynamics might bring these issues front and center. In order to sustain the relationship at healthy levels, it is necessary for the Submissive to be aware of and deal with whatever psychological issues they might have. This is a mutual thing as the Dominant will also have to deal with their issues while they deal with couple issues together. As they deal with their issues as individuals and as a couple, the d/s relationship also means finding a balance in which both partners can accept each other as they are. If one of the partners feels that being happy in the relationship would involve the other party changing their behavior radically, this is a recipe for failure.

Even though the Submissive confers upon the Dominant control of their selves, both partners are equally important to the relationship. Both partners choose the relationship because it works for them as they are. It has nothing to do with race, gender, sex or social standing. Preconceived prejudices on who is a suitable Dominant or Submissive are Subversive to the success of the relationship. The Submissive is not the inferior in the d/s relationship. Inferior and superior do not exist as concepts in the d/s world.

However, mistakes do happen like in any other relationship. Neither party is immune to messing up. This has to be understood by both parties going into the relationship and they can agree on ways to deal with it in advance. It has been known for Dominants to apologize to Submissives when they do something wrong. This is necessary to build a solid relationship based on trust. Even outside of normal human messing up, the Submissive is Subject to certain specific situations which might put extra pressure on them. Perhaps they find that they are unable to sustain the same level of pain play as they initially thought they might. Admitting to this might be hard for them to do because they perceive it as a being a failure as a Sub. However, they still need to deal with this or else they risk the relationship crumbling under the weight of too much expectation that might not gel with reality.

In order to avoid this and other problems, strong communication is key. This does not mean that the Submissive opens up to the Dom and the latter remains stoic. It is a two way street. The Submissive must examine their patterns of communication to make sure they are clear about their wants and needs and that they also hear what the Dom desires. They must be continually aware of the ways in which communication can improve and strive to enhance it. This is a constant trial for most people and it helps if they both accept that instead of looking at it as a chore. It is also essential to be aware how the different communication styles between Dom and Sub intersect and make sure they are effective.

There are boundaries within the d/s relationship. Just because one is a Submissive does not mean that they submit to everyone. The relationship might be strictly between the Submissive and their Dominant or they might have expected behavior within a community of d/s members. This is agree within the membership of that community or even between certain couples. So the Submissive might be expected to serve another Dominant within a circle the same way they do their own. This power dynamic is agreed upon within the individual d/s relationship rather than within the membership of a community.

It is essential to have outside support, however, because the intensity of the d/s relationship can be exhausting. It cannot exist in a vacuum and generally this is where the kink community comes in. It is a resource from which the Submissive can learn about relationship models which they can then customize to fit their own world view. Everyone in the community might have their own individualized concept of a certain kink but being able to discuss and learn and extrapolate is very helpful to self-discovery and awareness. Other ways to learn and grow as a Submissive includes reading materials, support and discussion groups, workshops and any number of books such as this one which give a framework to the lifestyle. It also helps to have friends with whom you can discuss issues that arise. A Submissive might have vanilla friends who can understand or offer a sympathetic ear but another Submissive would be able to understand the things that they go through the best.

If one partner doesn't wish the other to speak about the relationship to friends, this might be a sign that the relationship is unhealthy. It is important to make the distinction between being unable to ask for help or others' opinion and airing one's dirty laundry to all and sundry. The latter might be something any partner objects to but the former is a red flag. A wise Dominant should encourage and support the Submissive to seek counsel rather than restricting it.

It takes patience to get a relationship to the point of trust that can enable the Submissive to cede all control to the Dominant. The two people need to get to know each other well, and understand how each operates and what makes them tick. The Submissive needs to understand themselves and their needs and be able to communicate these clearly to their partner. They need to know what their limits are and understand that the boundaries to these limits are not static. They might change with

114

circumstances. The Dominant is the one who sets the pace but the Submissive must feel comfortable with the pace being set. There is all the time in the world to learn what pace is comfortable for both so rushing is unnecessary.

PART THREE

Action Plans

CHAPTER FIVE
Getting Started with the Lifestyle

O nce you've realized that you might have an interest in being a Submissive, knowing what to do next might be a challenge. That's where books like this and articles, podcasts, online communities come in. The first thing to realize, however, is that d/s play is free. It can be carried out any place at any time so long as you have a willing partner.

So as a matter of course, the first step is finding a willing partner. This might be easier said than done but there are a few hacks that you can use. The simplest is to simply post about it on your social media channels. Of course this might lead to some embarrassing interactions but being a Submissive is nothing to be ashamed of so if people want to troll you for it, that is absolutely their own boring, vanilla problem. Those that make fun of you are also helping by disqualifying themselves as possible matches. Once you've weeded these out, which might take an average of 48 hours before they lose interest, especially if you make a point not to be embarrassed about it, you can start to really screen your responses for interest. They very likely were part of your social circles already and once they see that you are interested, they will reach out to you.

Most people do follow some aspect of the d/s lifestyle and they are serious about it rather than having it as just a fun activity that they indulge in from time to time. Many people act Submissive at their jobs and to their bosses, they automatically obey rules given to them both by society and in their work environments. It's only the play aspects of d/s which is not so mainstream.

With the popularity of d/s clearly established, then you need to ask yourself; if you're ready to obey commands issued in your daily life without question well then why not take it further and really get to understand yourself by exploring aspects of your Submissiveness in play? At least that way, you get enjoyment out of it.

BDSM Meetup groups do exist in some cities and their quality differs from group to group. You can go to the group Meetup page for your city and if you like what you see you can see about attending a meeting. The chances are high that somebody you already know is in the lifestyle and would be interested in partnering with you if they knew that you were interested. It is understandable that some might want to keep this aspect of their personality a secret but that makes it more difficult to meet a good partner unless you are already associated with a d/s community.

Generally, a genuine interest in the lifestyle is nothing to hide or be ashamed of, and staying 'in the closet' only makes growth and maturity that much more difficult. However some communities might be close minded and the consequences of airing your interests might be severe. In this case, it is better to stay safe until such a time as you are able to express yourself without fear of actual bodily harm being done to you.

Another thing to avoid is trying to convince a person who has no interest in a d/s relationship to try it out with you. The lack of enthusiasm and interest is likely to kill that relationship even before it starts. The interested party will expend so much time and energy trying to explain, persuade or coerce that the experience loses its shine and the enjoyment goes out of it. Better to find someone who is already interested and enthusiastic about d/s and then you can both explore the ins and outs together. It is important to be patient, honest and steadfast when communicating with your partner about your needs. Allow the partner to agree to it or not and then go to the next step based on their answer. The worst thing to do is pretend disinterest because your partner is not agreeable to the lifestyle. Examine your options instead right from the possibility of ending the relationship to having an open relationship. Or you can turn your back on exploring d/s and live a vanilla lifestyle.

This might be easier if you have no experience of the lifestyle and therefore can genuinely say that you don't know what you're missing. Life is too short however to bury a part of yourself all for the sake of keeping an unsatisfactory relationship alive. Sooner or later, that type of situation ends in resentment.

CHAPTER SIX
Now that You've Found a Partner

N ow that you have searched for and found someone willing to explore the d/s lifestyle with you, what is next you ask? Well, it's always good to start with the basics, that is, letting the Dominant have control during sex. Power play is a broad concept and the scope of exploration is almost limitless. Before you decide to widen your horizons however, you must tackle the issue of safety.

Various books and Wikipedia entries might give you a clue as to what kind of Submissive you wish to be but each of these has risks. Seemingly uncomplicated acts such as spanking can turn hazardous if done too hard or on the wrong body part. Sometimes, just Googling on how to carry out a certain thing such as spanking, paddling, whipping safely and properly might give you the answers you seek. If you're using sex toys or props, make sure you both read the instructions thoroughly and maybe carry out a few taste tests before settling on a particular routine.

It is important to take it slow because the most important thing in d/s relationships, in any relationship really, is trust. And trust takes time to build.

Power dynamics not only have a physical element but also an emotional one. As a Submissive you will have to educate yourself on some of these dynamics so you're prepared when they come up and have formulated strategies on how to deal with them.

It is important to discuss boundaries and safe words with your Dominant. If you're using a checklist of items, go down each one by one and agree on limits, and just how far you're willing to go. Pick a safe word that normally would not come up in sexual or role play situations such as pineapple. When you as a Submissive utters the safe word, the Dom needs to stop immediately and conduct a check to see that everything is still fine.

The use of green, yellow and red signals great, fine but not really and stop immediately, respectively.

CHAPTER SEVEN
Ideas to Try

Role Play

This is a good way to ease into the lifestyle when you're still feeling awkward and unsure of yourself. Finding your inner Submissive might take time and effort and playing certain roles is a way of trying on different personas to see which one fits the best. It also gives you a script to follow when you might be feeling lost or overwhelmed. It might also be useful to use props such as costumes or equipment, which helps you get into the right mood. This is a way to get to know what your partner likes. Try not to take things too seriously; this should be fun so don't get too upset if either of you makes a mistake or even starts laughing. Common transformations for the Submissive include the sexy maid, student with a teacher, or Private taking orders from a Commander.

But it is entirely up to you to be as creative and outlandish as you wish. Is it not exciting to be regarded as perverted by a vanilla society? You might already have something in mind which you have been dying to try out and this is your time to go for it. Anything goes as long as you have discussed it with your partner, set your boundaries and refreshed yourselves about what the safe word is. Never humiliate your partner without warning or agreement and make them flounder so that they feel they can no longer trust you. Getting back to where you started might be extremely difficult or even impossible. That nanosecond of that feeling will definitely not be worth the weeks or months of trying to claw your way back into the glory of being adored, trusted and loved by the partner. Remember that whatever you do with or to your partner must be from a stance of adoration and love.

Below is a suggested role play scenario but of course each of us is unique. This is just to get you in the mood and give you ideas.

Poor Me (for the female)

You are a young woman who has just lost her job. You have just moved to the big city not long ago and have noone to call on for help. You are worried how to pay the rent on your apartment when the landlord calls this evening and you have to concoct a plan that might defer him evicting you. You dress in your sexiest of clothes: black stockings, a tie-up Basque, which ties under your breasts completely exposing them. You have high heels on and are wearing bright red lipstick and lots of mascara to make your eyes look as big as they can. You wear a see through negligee, which clearly shows your naked breasts and the tops of your stockings when you bend over just a little bit. You open a bottle of wine while you wait for the landlord to arrive. Right on time, there is a knock on the door and you go to answer it.

"Oh, there you are, Mr. Henderson. Please come in. I'm sorry I'm not properly dressed. I was just getting ready for a bath."

"That's quite all right Lizzie. I'm liking what I see."

"Would you like a glass of wine? I have something I have to talk to you about."

"I don't mind if I do Lizzie. You're the last on my rounds." Bend over to get out a glass and so that he can see your pants and everything else your thong reveals.

"What is it you want to discuss Lizzie?"

"Well, the thing is Mr. Henderson that I've lost my job."

"Oh dear, does that mean you will be leaving?"

"Well, I was hoping we might be able to reach some arrangement. That I might be able to pay you in another way."

"And what would that be Lizzie?" Stand up and drop your negligee to show your breasts. Offer one of them up to him.

"Would you like some of this, Mr. Henderson?"

"Well that looks very nice, but I think I'll be needing a bit more than that. In fact, I think that you're a very naughty girl to expect me to suck on your tit in place of the rent. Perhaps I should spank you to teach you a lesson."

"Yes, Mr. Henderson, I know I deserve it. I think you should."

"And after that, I think that you should suck my dick. Do you agree to my terms so far?"

"Yes, Mr. Henderson."

"Come here." Walk over to him and he puts you over his knees and spanks you. He will then take out his dick and you must suck it. When he is ready, he will bend you over and take you in any position he likes.

"Now Lizzie. That was payment for this week. I will be back next week at the same time, okay?"

"Yes, Mr. Henderson."

"Okay."

"Is that all you have to say Lizzie. I think I deserve a bit more than that for my understanding don't you?"

"Thank you, Mr. Henderson."

"That's better. And in future, I'd appreciate it if you call me Sir. Okay?"

"Yes, sir. Thank you, sir."

Please Don't Fire Me (for the male)

You are the only man working in a firm of financial consultants. The only other employees are all female as is your boss, a very sexy lady who terrifies you because she is so confident and bossy. You try not to meet her eyes because she always picks fault with you and makes you feel little. You go into the office one day and there is no one else there but you need to get a report done for one of your customers that you are seeing tomorrow. Your boss is in her office and it is quite late and already dark outside. You are at your computer and she comes and calls you into her office.

"Frampton – get here. Now!"

"Yes, Ms. Filly. Is there something I can do for you?"

"Now, it's funny that you should ask that Frampton. Because there is indeed something you can do for me. Come in and shut the door. Don't sit down. Stand there." She points with a ruler or a pen.

"Well, I suppose if that's all that on offer today, I'll have to take advantage of it. I suppose it's better than nothing. Strip off….. What are you staring at? Strip! Now! Take everything off. I want to see everything."

"But Ms. Filly, this is sexual harassment, there are laws against this."

"Shut up, Frampton. I am your boss but I won't be for long if you don't do exactly as I say. Is that understood?"

136

"Yes, Ms. Filly."

"And I want you to call me Mistress. Do you understand? And I don't just mean today. You will always call me Mistress from now. Even in front of your workmates."

"Yes, Mistress."

"And you're going to do as you're told?"

"Yes, Mistress."

"Good boy. Now strip. Now!"

You remove all of your clothes and stand in front of her naked. She snorts.

"Are you married, Frampton?"

"Yes, Mistress."

"And how the hell do you keep your wife happy?"

"She seems happy Mistress."

"She's kidding you. Come round here."

She pulls up her skirt to reveal that she is wearing stockings and no panties.

"On your knees. Show me how you make your wife happy. I'm thinking that you must have a very clever tongue. Put your tongue out and let me see it. Well yeah, now put that between my legs and make me come."

You do as she orders.

"Not bad, now lick it all out. I am so wet. Good boy. Now over my desk please. I am going to give you something to remember."

You bend over her desk and she ties your hands behind your back. You feel her part your ass cheeks and she is rubbing oil into your anus with her finger. She inserts a vibrator into your ass and starts it going. When it has been

138

going for a little while, and you are really enjoying yourself, she starts to paddle your ass just below the vibrator. You were not expecting it and the shock makes you shout out.

"Silence! You little toad. For that, you are not having the pleasure of the vibrator. You don't deserve it. And don't you dare come."

She continues to paddle your ass until you think you can't take anymore and suddenly then she stops. She inserts a butt plug up your ass.

"Stand up slug!"

You stand up and she takes your place. She pulls up her skirt and parts her legs wide.

"Fuck me toad! As hard as you can. And you had better make me come."

When you have made her come she stands up and straightens her skirt.

"Not too bad for the first time. Get dressed and get on with your work."

"Yes, Mistress." You dress and leave the office as she calls out to you,

"Oh and Toad, you will do that whenever I demand it. Do you understand?"

"Yes, Mistress. And do not take out the butt plug until you leave the office."

"Yes, Mistress."

"What do you say to me?"

"Thank you, Mistress."

"You are ready to obey me?"

"Yes, Mistress. Thank you."

You leave the office.

Cuckolding

This can only be practiced if both partners agree to it. Obviously, there are different combinations but normally it is the women who performs sex with another man. This may be in front of the man or with his knowledge at least. The partner may be allowed to join in or he might have to sit in the room and watch his partner having sex. Alternatively, this might be with another woman, which would seem to resonate with a lot of men's fantasies, and really not a punishment for anyone. More unusual is the scenario when the man has another woman. This might be the case if the man's partner does not want an S&D relationship and the wife agrees that he can see a professional dominatrix. Alternatively, it might be a threesome where another woman is invited to join the couple. The female partner might have to perform sex acts on the other woman such as sucking her breasts or licking her pussy, generally getting her ready for her partner. Maybe she could shave her pubes and massage her or spank her. Another scenario is when the couple uses the third person as a domestic and a sex slave or the female is used for a gang bang scenario while her partner watches. At the end, he is verbally abusive to her using her for sex himself, in any way he chooses.

Group sex or cuckolding can be with a stranger or someone that is the friend of both of them. However, be very careful who you choose to join you as if S&D is included this might be an unknown quantity and expose you to danger. You should also draw up very firm boundaries that you both agree should definitely not be crossed. Within a loving partnership, sharing your partner with someone else can be a mark of true respect for them. You trust them to come back to you because you love them but you want others to share appreciate your partner's body and remind yourself that you are their owner and their body belongs to you. It is your property to lend out as you please.

Going to a BDSM Club

Because this type of practice is becoming more prevalent in society, the entrepreneurs amongst us are learning how to exploit it and provide a venue for enthusiasts to meet. The clubs are pretty upbeat and if you decide you want to visit one take your time to choose an outfit. Everybody dresses up so be inventive to make the best of your experience. You are likely to meet some pretty way out characters but there will be lots of interesting people and you will be able to pick up a fair few new ideas. These places usually have playrooms that are set up like BDSM rooms so if you go into it. Be prepared to see men and women dressed up in an array of costumes and being subjected to various levels of punishment. You are likely to see individuals wearing collars, which denote that they belong to someone else and

143

some of these collars will have leads attached to them and will be led by another person. Some people might even have more than one pet attached to leads. It is certainly an eye opener but should be titillating too.

The only thing that you should be aware of is that there are people of all persuasions who frequent these places so you might run into gay men or lesbians, subs, domes, or any combination thereof. There will also be singles and couples and perhaps threesomes or more. You're bound to find someone on your wavelength who likes the same things as you do, but of course, that doesn't necessarily mean you have to join in.

Bondage

When it comes to power dynamics, nothing says loss of all control like being tied up. The Dominant has all the power in their hands once they have you trussed up like a chicken and for you to be comfortable in that situation takes a lot of trust. When just starting out, you can use the sport sheets under the bed restraint system or Velcro straps which are easily removed. If you have ever seen Fifty Shades of Grey or read the book, you will already be familiar with the degrees of bondage (shades, of course) which can be implemented. Obviously, you might not want to go to such extremes as having a dungeon in your basement but you could equip a spare room, or even your bedroom, quite easily so that it includes equipment, which can be hidden away easily, maybe from the prying eyes of your home help or your mother in law. There are also less dramatic ways of creating an atmosphere of bondage, and just by simply securing your partner's limbs and using the appropriate body language sends out a feeling of sexual power that makes the other person feel vulnerable.

It can be enormously liberating to be tied up because the decision for doing all of the naughty things you have constantly been told you shouldn't be doing is taken out of your hands. Even though you enjoy it, that little voice keeps telling you that this is be forbidden. But what choice do you have? Your partner has you tied up or has just spanked you so you have to submit and do as he says. And enjoy yourself into the bargain. It can be extremely erotic to be spanked by your partner and be dominated so that you can easily pretend that you are being forced to do something and that someone has complete power over you to make you do so.

This might be especially exciting if the submissive were to wear a sexual aid that could be remotely controlled by a partner in public. If a person does not comply with their partner's wishes, the remote device can be operated to give an electrical impulse that can either be used to instigate a direct sexual response or a shock applied to the genitals. Either scenario can send out the message of Wait until I get you home and then both partners are sexually excited all the evening and cannot wait to leave.

It can be especially erotic if one of you is spanked is front of another person or people and then every time you see them again, you are reminded of that instance and that they saw your bare ass and whatever else they might be able to spot. It is certainly going to make their night and probably your partner's. Have fun trying.

Feminization/Sissy Play

This is making the man dress up as a woman and act like a woman. He might wear make-up and the couple either just keep it to themselves around the house or he might go out in public dressed up as a woman. Forced feminization is quite different to the man who wants to cross-dress. Forced feminization is when he is not given a choice and is ordered to do so by the woman. It is performed for the enjoyment of the woman and she might make him look at himself in a full-length mirror or force him to go out in public. The woman might even then use a strap-on dildo and fuck him forcing him to watch in a mirror or she could set up a camera to film it and make him watch it afterward while playing with his penis.

Talk

The power dynamic can be played up using terms such as master or mistress or sir to refer to the Dominant. Polite phrasing like please and thank you is used by the Submissive when the Dominant does something for them and they use deferential language when addressing the Dom. Language can also be used when the couple is in bed or in public, which can be degrading to the other person. This can either be said in front of other people so that they can hear or in lowered tones, but so that the quiet conversation is noticed by others. For instance, as a

148

prelude to sex, one partner could call the other derogative names such as slut, whore or worm. Even during sex, one could say to the other something like, Do you like that, slut? You are so good to ride. I am going to fuck you until your eyes pop, bitch. This sort of language could be used as a whisper in public or on a journey on a train or in a restaurant. The other person should be deferential and reciprocate saying that they can't wait. Language can also be used for phone sex so that someone could call or text dirty language to the other. Erotic poetry can also be employed to turn the other person on. Try and write something yourself and make it specific to your partner.

Asking Permission

The Submissive asks permission of the Dominant before doing anything in the bedroom. This emphasizes that the Submissive is there to serve and to please. The Submissive might plead for the chance to kiss or caress the Dom. They might not orgasm before the Dom gives them permission to. Sometimes the Submissive will not even touch themselves before the Dom says they can. If they do something without asking for permission then the Dom may have to dole out punishment until the sub is trained properly to know their place. If they still do not obey completely, then the punishment gets harsher.

This could also be used for simple things like asking if you are allowed go out socializing with your friends. Permission may only be given if some kind of chastity device is worn by the person going out and maybe a butt plug is required too.

Permission could be sought also to have sex with someone else and this might be agreed but only if they are going to be told about the sex in great detail. It might also involve some sort of punishment or a photograph showing the woman sucking the other man's dick.

Permission can be sought from the other partner for simple masturbation. This might be agreed if the other partner is allowed to watch or perhaps to join in with a vibrator perhaps.

Strap-On Play

If this is his first time, then you will have to take it easy to start with. You have to start stretching him and use lots of lubrication. Try putting some lubrication on your finger and using that to start with. You can wear latex gloves if you wish. When you have stretched him a little you can start using long thin butt plugs and progress up to something a bit fatter for a strap-on dildo. Always use lubrication. You can either take him bending over something or if you want to see his face as you're doing it, get him to lie flat with his legs bent up. This makes the man feel extremely vulnerable and at your mercy so is very powerful tool in male submission. It will also make you

151

feel extremely powerful and really help you get into your dominant role. Because this is highly physical, take things slowly and be sure that you use the safe word if it is needed. And ask him what he liked about it afterward or if there is anything that he did not like.

Punishments

Of course, if there are things that are forbidden, that require permission, it also means that there are consequences to disobedience. If the Submissive touches themselves without permission the Dom might punish them with a spanking or refusing to touch them for a stated period of time. Infractions and punishments should be discussed beforehand to make sure that both parties are comfortable with the extent to which they are going. The power dynamic is a very delicate thing which needs to be handled with care.

You should always discuss what type of punishment will be invoked before each session. This doesn't have to be in great detail but what might have been acceptable in the previous session, or at least which the sub accepted, may no longer be acceptable in the next one. The sub may not have wanted to spoil the moment so submitted to it. but if they are completely repulsed by it, and say that they do not want to submit to it again, then their wishes should be respected. You should always remind yourselves of the safe word before every session. Never ignore that safe word because by doing so, you are breaking all ethics and destroying your partner's trust and faith in you.

There are sadists who enjoy inflicting real pain on other people, including their partners. This is where sadism/masochism differs from sub/dom relationships. Within the latter, punishment is meted out within a loving relationship and can actually serve as a healing process. When a person gives themselves over to another person, it is sometimes to work through things that have happened in the past and resolve them. It's not just about the physical side of domination but involves discussion with your loved one and after a session is over, the couple will cuddle and discuss what has happened during the session. With sadism/masochism, sex is not necessarily within a loving relationship and can be quite cold and cruel. Be quite clear about the difference. People who enjoy hurting others physically or mentally can be psychopathic and need treatment for a medical condition which they might be unable to control. An S&D relationship should ideally be enacted within a loving relationship so that it is a healing process as well as one of total confidence in another person.

The Pain Factor

The amount of pain any Submissive is willing to undergo varies with each individual. As seen in part one, the levels of pain go from one to six and each one has its own characteristics. To understand one's pain tolerance requires a lot of trial and error with a Dom you can trust. Make sure to start small, with some spanking, slapping, pulling of hair, choking and pinching before upping the ante. Even at its mildest, however, it is important that you stay safe. This means getting educated on the right way to play these games. However, pain is an important part of S&D and combined with sexual actions can provide erotic and exquisite pain. This is probably an extension of having your power taken away from you. By being out of control and handing any power or responsibility over to your partner, you are abdicated from feeling any guilt because you have no choice but to take part in the forbidden activities so you can relax and enjoy them. The pain does not have to be excruciating but it probably has to be so hard that it is convincing. If it isn't then it cannot be sufficiently harsh as to destroy the guilt that may be inhibiting you from have a truly liberated sex life. The level of pain does not necessarily have to equate to the level of guilt however. The level of pain must always depend on the level that the sub is capable of sustaining.

Sex Toys

The selection of accessories available to enhance the d/s power play is wide and varied. Experimenting is always fun, especially with new things. A new Sub might start with relatively vanilla items like blindfolds and handcuffs, graduate to ball gags or nipple clamps and even try spreader bars. For punishments and funishments there are always whips, chains and paddles. Butt plugs are fairly ubiquitous for Submissives of both sexes as well as cock cages, chastity belts and other reminders of ownership such as collars. Different costumes can be added to enhance the play portion of the game. There is tons of stuff online and it can be fun looking together or alternatively surprising your partner. If you have any fetishes such as wearing rubber or PVC then this sort of clothing is now readily available. As mentioned in a previous part of the book, remotely controlled electronic toys are enormous fun too and can be used erotically to emphasize control of your partner in public places. It serves as a reminder of who is the dom and who is the sub. Toys needn't all be items of punishment. For instance, dildos and vibrators can be used to give pleasure rather than punishment. And even the proverbial forms of punishment and torture are actually giving pleasure at some level. It depends on perspective and it might seem strange but it is possible that someone can actually look forward to a spanking or another form of pain depending on the circumstances and environment, and obviously who is administering it.

Expanding to Outside the Bedroom

Once the Submissive is comfortable within the relationship in the sexual sphere, it's time to expand outside of that area and attempt to live the d/s lifestyle in other areas. It does not mean being a 24/7 Submissive, it is easier if you take things slowly. You might start by agreeing on certain hours or days when you are in play mode, and then using the 'off' days to recover or process the experience.

During the play hours, the Submissive is bound to follow certain guidelines as set up by the Dom and agreed to by the Sub. This includes things they must do and things they can't do without permission. Other things are outright forbidden. For example, they might be expected to address the Dom as sir/madam, or master/mistress at all times without fail. They might be forbidden to touch themselves in a sexual way unless the Dom says they can. They may not orgasm without permission. Sometimes they are forbidden to orgasm at all.

If they fail to adhere to these strictures then they are Subject to punishment. If the infraction is light, the punishment might actually be something the Submissive enjoys such as paddling or wearing a butt plug for short periods. As the infractions become more serious, the punishments also become more pain filled. The Submissive might be asked to wear the plug for days, or kneel in the corner facing away from the Dom, or forbidden to orgasm for a week. They might take the form of chores.

Sometimes a couple's work life can dictate how S&D is introduced into the relationship. If the woman works longer hours than the man, for instance, it might be necessary that the man has to take a more active role in the housework and childcare. This can happen quite naturally over time and often does not even require negotiation.

One partner might offer to do this because it is practical but also because they want to help their partner and ensure the work is evenly spread. This shows their loving and caring side and the other person feels cared for and appreciated. Gradually this behavior works its way into areas of the couple's lives such as childcare and the person who takes the sub role receives sexual or other types of favors from their now dominant partner. The male might bring his partner flowers or take her out for fancy meals. He might emphasize his dominance by spanking her and making her dress in an ultra-feminine fashion. The female may make her male sub service her orally or she may spank him or deny him orgasms. There are many kinds of differences on a theme and it is up to the couple to discover how creative that they can be.

Once the Submissive is sure that the lifestyle is for them, they might enter into a long term contract with a Dominant to live the lifestyle 24/7.

The main thing with the d/s relationship is to always have the channels of communication open so they both parties can be reassured constantly that they are happy with the bond as is and they are staying safe. As important as the play sessions are, the aftercare where the Dom wraps the Sub up in blankets and cuddles them and takes care of them. This is the time when they debrief each other on how satisfactory the session was and keep each other clued in on their emotional state.

Discussing what actually occurred immediately after the session is not only necessary to dissect what is and what was not to be repeated and to measure acceptable levels of pain, but it can be quite an erotic turn on too. For instance, one might say to the other, 'I loved it when you put your finger in my ass. It made me want to come immediately.' Doing this may precipitate into another session because the feelings are so powerful. This can be especially true if the couple likes to indulge in sex talk, either face to face or on the phone or email.

Human Ashtray

This might be on the wane in popularity as more people give up smoking but the submissive is used as an ashtray. This is not to the point that the cigarette is stubbed out on them but the sub might collect the ash in their hand or even on their tongues. It could even be flicked onto an exposed area of their bodies.

Human Furniture

The sub might kneel down on all fours and the dom puts their feet across their back to use them as a footstool. The sub might be in a state of undress or be partially dressed.

Swinging Parties

This is where partners are swapped on a regular basis. Men put their car keys in a receptacle so that all car keys are together. All the men take turns at removing a set of keys each and the keys that correspond with the key holder's wife/partner has sex with the person who chose the key. This used to be seen as being more beneficial to the man because the woman was more likely to have feelings of feeling used whereas the man feels more dominant because he is the gender who is responsible for choosing the key. In reality, this practice can be extremely erotic for the woman as well and, once alone, the couple might practice S&D where the woman takes the dominant role. It all adds to the excitement because no one can be sure who they are going to have sex with at all. This type of sex could be used in S&D between a couple because it could be conceived as a male or female allowing their property to be used by someone else and only because they have given their consent. It might be like a pride of lions having indiscriminate sex while the choice is removed from the woman and she must do as she is told.

Public Sexual Object

This might be at a sex party when there is a choice of sexual activities to join in. There might be a couple having various types of sex while watched by an audience. This could be full sex or spanking or oral sex. It could be two women or two men. The dominant partner offers his sub up for this type of sexual degradation. It could also involve tying their naked or semi-naked partner down and inviting other party guests to use them as they wish. This might involve fucking and could entertain a couple when the male fucks the female and the female gets her to satisfy her orally. To heighten excitement she could also be blindfolded so she is unaware who is actually using her.

164

She could be filmed and at the next party, the film is shown to add further degradation. The man then fucks his partner in front of others to the cheers of everyone present. If all party guests consist of couples where the man is dominant and the woman is submissive, this is even better because all women must submit to any man telling them what to do. By the very fact that the couple is at the party, they are agreeing to this. The male dresses his partner up and when she removes her coat, she might be naked apart from stockings and high heels. In fact, every woman could be made to remove her coat in front of the others. One person wins the green ticket, which means that man gets to have as many women as he can manage. Women who are not as subservient as any of the man present desires is sent to him to be spanked publically by him and then made to suck his dick. There can often be an age difference so that a young girl ends up with an old man or a young man ends up with a woman in her sixties. Of course, the men have the right to refuse but the women do not. If a man refuses her, she becomes the sympathy fuck for anyone who wants a go and can manage another fuck. Another version is that all the women bend over in a line, maybe on all fours so that they feel extra submissive. The men move along the line, fucking each one in turn. If they prefer, they can move to the other side and have the woman suck their dick.

Prostitution

This can be used when the man thinks that the woman needs to be taught a lesson and he arranges to sell her to anyone who will pay. He might invite his friends to watch him shave her pussy first and then he charges a nominal fee of say $10 each for his friends or strangers to fuck his partner. When they have all had a go, he spanks her and goes out for a drink after tying her to the bed to wait for when he gets back. Alternatively, he might play a game of cards for her and the winner of each round gets to fuck her.

He might be in the same room to make sure that she is in no danger and the men queue up outside the bedroom door to wait their turn. If he is not in the room, he could have a camera set up or there could be a two-way mirror so that the men who are waiting their turn could watch each other enjoying themselves.

Erotic Humiliation

Quite a few of the above activities fall under this category. With the advent of the Internet this can be worldwide and not just kept to a few. It might not be about the money when a man exploits his woman through sex. He might get her to do phone sex for strangers who ring up and pay her to speak dirty to them until they come. She might feel degraded or humiliated by this but it reminds her that he is in charge of her and she is in no real danger, especially because it is anonymous. Another version might be to use a webcam so that strangers can see her touching her breasts or see her wriggling naked. She might have to use a vibrator on herself or masturbate using her own hand. She might have to suck her partner's dick, but only she would be in-camera, not her partner, unless he wants to be of course. Of course, this can only be done with the female's agreement, but it can prove to be highly erotic, and sex with her partner afterwards can be amazing when she thinks about a load of faceless strangers looking at her body or see her performing sexual acts. If she is not totally convinced or comfortable, then she doesn't have to show her face. Just by showing her body to a faceless public can arouse her sufficiently to make her want to keep doing it. This could stretch to putting on a show for a private paying audience. This could be by stripping or pole dancing and then stripping off totally and letting a selecting person fuck her. Or it might be saying that she is a life model for photographers and advertising where it is likely to attract a lot of men – or women – who are actually not photographically inclined. You should discuss beforehand whether your partner is in agreement with appearing in publications for those who will pay for erotic photos. It could easily happen that you open up a magazine and see your partner displayed in all her exposed wonder. How are you both going to feel? Be sure that this is something that you both want.

Exchanging roles

What happens when the student overtakes the master? What if the student wants to flip roles? As you become more and more sexually self aware your inhibitions will fall away and you will be on a journey to further sexual freedom. As you manage to overcome everything that has held you back one inhibition at a time, your boundaries will stretch and you will realize that there are so many things yet to discover. You have lived your life so far in a cocoon cushioned away from real fulfillment. It might seem that

169

the more you know, the more you need to know but you are embarking on a remarkable journey that can only provide sexual enlightenment and fulfillment. Embrace it. You might never have considered being the dominant partner but perhaps this has always been a major sexual dream of your partner. As you go further along the path of sexual self- discovery, your boundaries may well relax and you will find yourself agreeing to something that you might not have even vaguely considered six months ago. All at once, you will discover you are a different person. Your partner might raise the courage to tell you that he/she wants to be dominated and controlled, which means your deeply ingrained roles must be reversed or at least challenged. You have been used to being the sub so it might be a huge challenge to flip into a dominant role. Where do you go from here? You love your partner; you know that. You want to please them; that's a definite. Okay, so the first thing you do is research it. Look up every article you can find on the Internet. Grab hold of every magazine and book on the subject. Look at YouTube guides. Join a support group where there are others in the same position as you. Perhaps every nerve in your body is telling you to reject the demand but your heart is telling you that at the very least you should try to comply. But what you should be doing as a very definite requirement is communicating. Ask them why they want to do this and why are they suddenly suggesting it? Maybe they have been harboring this desire for so long and this is exactly the way you can totally satisfy them. You might be averse to the suggestion at first but if you love your partner then the very least you can do is try it because this might be the fundamental turning point in your sex life. This will have a knock on effect on your lives on a wider scale too as your axis reverses and shakes up your world.

Verbal Punishment

Insults can be just as powerful as using physical punishment. Before implementing this though, agree between you that you are in role-play mode. Let them be under no misapprehension that what you are saying might be true and your genuine thoughts. If they should believe that what you are saying is, in fact true, obviously this could have severe detrimental repercussions on your relationship.

Conversely, language can be employed to spice up actions. For instance, a female domme could employ insults to use in her role with the male sub to subjugate his will to hers. A suggested use of such language might be as follows.

"What is that, you sniveling little worm? Or is it a sniveling little worm?"

"It's my dick mistress."

"What! I've never seen such a poor excuse for a dick. And what do you intend to do with that worm?"

"Anything my mistress commands. I am here to please you."

"And you think that you can please me with that? I suspect that we might need something much bigger than that to please me, don't you worm?"

"I'll try my best, mistress."

"Your best? What good is that? I need something much bigger. Perhaps I will have to find someone else with a big dick to fuck me. Would you like to watch that worm?"

"Yes, mistress."

"And then I will make you like his sperm out of me. Would you like that worm?"

"Yes, mistress."

"How much would you like it, worm? Very much? If you would, get on your knees and kiss my feet. Now!"

Worm does as he is commanded.

So you get the picture.

It is up to you if you have this conversation face to face or by telephone when your partner is at work or in a room full of strangers although it would be especially difficult for him to explain why he is calling the person on the phone mistress. But that might even add to the erotic nature of the language.

Verbal punishment can be administered by refusing to speak to the partner. Issue a command and if they ask for clarity or when they can stop, hit him across the face or on the butt or even whip them. Tell them at the start of the session that they is not allowed to speak and if they do, then they will have to suffer the consequences, which you must always carry through. They could be locked in a room for instance and left in solitary confinement while you go out with your friends for a meal. Tell them that they must be ready to service you when you get back but that you do not wish to hear any complaints or hear their sniveling. If they do object, their punishment and confinement period will be doubled.

CONCLUSION
Tips to Remember

Being a Submissive can be hot and fun; it's also a great way to do some self-exploration and discover new facets of your sexuality. Many people assume that Submissiveness is about doing as you're told but as we have seen, there are many types of Submissives and you can find the type that fits you.

You don't have to pile on the pressure on yourself. Above all, you should be having fun otherwise what is the point? Relax and let whatever happens happen. Putting pressure on yourself to be the perfect Submissive or to endure levels of pain you're not ready for means that both you and your Dominant will end up having a horrible time and the beauty of the experience is lost.

Sometimes simple is best; especially in the beginning. Sometimes all you need is the right words to catapult you into the scene. Yes, there is a place for whips and chains, but sometimes all you need is, "Don't come until I give you permission" to put you in the right mood.

Experimentation is where it's at. Try out different looks and different toys to get you in the right head space.

Sometimes just having a discussion with your Dominant is enough to get you all hot and bothered. Role playing with words might be enough to get you going to such an extent as you achieve gratification on words alone. Role playing with words is also an excellent way to learn each other's triggers and tells and enhances communication between you.

Get inspired by your favorite movies and shows. Fifty Shades of Grey has inspired many to be more honest about their d/s needs. But just being the Khaleesi and his sun and stars might be what you need to get you going.

You might twist the normal clichéd roles and take them in unexpected directions. For example when role playing doctor and patient, you might switch roles so that the Dom is the patient and the Sub is the doctor and so all the power is in the patient's hands. This opens up a new vista of possibilities about where to take the role play. It keeps the games fresh and new.

During after care and down time as a Submissive, you can process your experiences and really come to an appreciation of which ones really make you hot and bothered and which ones are just okay. This helps you to get to know yourself better. It's a learning process and when both Dom and Sub are invested, they can take their relationship to new heights simply by continuously refining what they know about each other and themselves. As the relationship becomes closer, it might become less necessary to articulate every desire; the Submissive might know immediately when they are out of line and what punishment is next. It makes the d/s play more seamless and reduces the amount of 'downtime' needed.

You can take advantage of occasions in the vanilla world that require dressing up in costumes to play up your d/s relationship and add more spice by being public about your lifestyle while still being decorous because everyone is dressed in costumes. Occasions such as Halloween or fancy dress parties are perfect for a different kind of role play that satisfies an exhibitionist kink you might have.

REFERENCES

https://pdfcrowd.com//genpdf/77fce6562f611bfe0e0bc52c
8e6bdfd4.pdf?name=www_rewriting_the_rules_co
m_sex_Dominant_and_Submissive_rela.pdf

https://pdfcrowd.com//genpdf/27b09a6ec7f6c53619a8036
6f598096c.pdf?name=aSubmissivesinitiative_wordp
ress_com_2013_04_20_being_a_Subm.pdf

https://pdfcrowd.com//genpdf/30060ca3fd1c97b28303c85
497487b4e.pdf?name=Submissivecircle_com_rights
_and_responsibilities.pdf

https://pdfcrowd.com//genpdf/989623a373c02b21d8c847
72473c26d2.pdf?name=www_huffingtonpost_com
_sandra_lamorgese_phd_Submissive_sex_p.pdf

https://pdfcrowd.com//genpdf/c737a3318edeaee14439de0
8dc7346c1.pdf?name=www_marieclaire_com_sex_l
ove_advice_a7422_Submissive_sex_con.pdf

https://pdfcrowd.com//genpdf/d5828c731baa850d94ee221
50b5c522f.pdf?name=friskybusinessboutique_com_
the_endorphin_levels_in_bdsm.pdf

https://pdfcrowd.com//genpdf/62ba2b6c44de99930cf90b9
68ee53ca9.pdf?name=www_kinkweekly_com_artic
le_baadmaster_slave_vs_Submissive.pdf

https://pdfcrowd.com//genpdf/afb1e92129f72d2c932baa7
c9889a8e7.pdf?name=growinguplittle_wordpress_c
om_2013_02_07_daddy_Doms_little_g.pdf

https://pdfcrowd.com//genpdf/c20e5c7d2a51ce8e273e0e6
0ce85523a.pdf?name=www_kinkly_com_definition
_6753_sissy_training.pdf

https://pdfcrowd.com//genpdf/9a7ee4771ad499b2427e2ae
be154c260.pdf?name=www_scribd_com_doc_5147
6645_The_Brat_Sub.pdf

https://pdfcrowd.com//genpdf/a9987af92bddff70b77094b
108878426.pdf?name=Dominantguide_com_1525_t
he_brat_ownership_guide.pdf

https://pdfcrowd.com//genpdf/eefaf5e759eaa8f15e417a8af
d16c4a4.pdf?name=sexgeek_wordpress_com_2010_
07_08_10_principles_for_healthy_2.pdf

https://pdfcrowd.com//genpdf/caa4ad2ad20fd7f657572ad
099532e69.pdf?name=www_yourtango_com_2013
186493_why_being_Submissive_relationsh.pdf

https://pdfcrowd.com//genpdf/1bf5de4a604e69cc6c3ceb6
713215d38.pdf?name=www_bustle_com_articles_1
21087_8_ways_to_be_Submissive_in_be.pdf

https://pdfcrowd.com//genpdf/b03f3fd742dee28c31fdd65
05e32ff0f.pdf?name=eprogressiveportfolio_blogspo
t_co_ke_2012_06_normal_0_false_.pdf

https://pdfcrowd.com//genpdf/a8c43515b5f7f9b766c04a3
784521ac1.pdf?name=www_buzzfeed_com_annabo
rges_role_play_tips_utm_term_vwGK7Bvv.pdf

Preview of Dominant Women: The Dominant Women's and Submissive Men's Handbook For Amazing Relationships

Introduction

The concept of dominance and submission is viewed as anathema in vanilla society. Most people don't understand how one can relish being submissive to another or give up that kind of control and trust another human being with your body like that. It is viewed as an outdated concept, and that's when the dominant is male and the submissive is female. The idea that a man might want to be the submissive is just inviting ridicule and disbelief.

Unfortunately, the benefits that bondage provides in a relationship with two consenting adults is often overlooked or simply not understood. So let us start from the beginning and define what dominance and submission mean. In the simplest terms, domination and submission refer to a power exchange between two consenting adults. The division between who is submissive and who is dominant is not limited by age, sex or gender. The level of domination and submission varies within relationships. In some it is limited solely to the bedroom, in others it carries on to other household dynamics. In very few of these relationships, it is a full lifestyle with the dominant making all decisions with total power control.

In what might be surprising to most people, the most common type of submission is male submission. This has been illustrated in erotic fiction and film, due to the appeal of thumbing a nose at the patriarchy. The domination of these males might be psychological or sexual in nature;

186

being required to please their dominant before they are allowed to achieve arousal. In other cases, orgasm is denied until the dominant says they can come. This could be arbitrary or based upon certain behavior or completion of certain tasks.

Because it is traditional for males to dominate a relationship, flipping it and reversing it so that the female takes the Domme role can be sexually liberating and also very arousing. Since the act of sex usually involves inserting the phallus into the vagina, the male is often considered as the 'active' partner. The phallus actively penetrates the submissive vagina and so the latter is considered to be receptive. This leads to males fantasizing about male chastity in a bid to subvert this notion. It arouses them to relinquish control because they are expected to always be in control. To expound on this, it must be reiterated that the submissive does not submit by force. They willingly surrender all their power to the dominant. This can be a difficult concept to understand in that in a paradoxical way, the act of submitting and surrendering all power to the dominant is an act of dominance within your submission. The submissive always have a safe word, which they can use to immediately stop any activity they are tired of, are not in agreement with or would simply like to discontinue.

If the submissive feels unsafe, threatened, uncomfortable or scared by anything going on they invoke the safe word. It's their security blanket, which ensures that they will never be forced to do anything they don't want to or which is beyond their comfort levels or safety. This shows that the submissive is actually the one with all the power in the relationship because they have an emergency exit button that they can use at any time.

This book will look at the male submissive in a heterosexual relationship with a female Domme. As was mentioned earlier, this relationship might take place only in the bedroom or extend to everyday household activities. Male submission can also take place in a dungeon, with a professional Domme, using role play that is usually non-sexual in nature.

Research has shown that many high profile individuals faced with tough daily decisions at work where they are placed in high stakes dominant positions find sexual and psychological relief by being submissive in their relationships. The submissive role is stress relieving and liberating for them because they are constantly in charge of every aspect of their professional lives and give that control up in their sexual relationship. When they give up their power in this way, they not only relieve stress but it is also beneficial to them and their lifestyles.

Steve Jobs and Mark Zuckerberg have done interviews in which they both admit to wearing similar outfits on a daily basis in order to take away that one decision from the myriad ones they have to make every day. This helps them to focus on other things that matter more and helps them to do their jobs better.

In choosing submission, the man relinquishes his power in one way while still retaining it in all others. The use of a safe word enables them to have peace of mind as they willingly put their well being in someone else's hands. They are able to explore and bring to life their sexual fantasies and erotic thoughts without fear. Being able to do this is far from being helpless or powerless contrary to popular belief. This book will seek to debunk all the myths behind male submission and take a deep dive into what it means.

PART ONE: BEING A DOMINANT WOMAN

I t might be difficult trying to remember when your sexuality was first awakened and how you felt. Similarly, it might be difficult remembering that first realization that you wanted to adopt the role of being a dominant woman, specifically sexually. Slowly, it dawns on you that vanilla sex might never be quite enough to satisfy you completely. Perhaps it was someone else who introduced you to this lifestyle and you realized how much more this extra dimension brought into your life. But when the relationship ended, new partners never had that same sexual proclivity and so you let it lie but thought you would never be fully satisfied again. So you resigned

191

yourself to that fact and waited for someone else to come along and to light your fire. And then, you find someone who you are totally in love with and you settle down into marriage, never having discussed this desire because you feel embarrassed or a little afraid that he might think you're a freak.

Stop right there! If you are so in love with a guy that you are going to commit to him for life, then you need to discuss your innermost thoughts and make sure that you both trust each other with your lives and each other's body. If you commit to a life of vanilla sex without even exploring the options and keeping your mouth firmly shut, then you could potentially be signing up for a lifetime of boring and unfulfilling sex. And committing your poor husband to be to a wife who he feels he can never satisfy sexually. So you need at least to discuss what turns you both on. Yes, of course he might be a bit stunned at first never suspecting his cute little angel could have anything quite so hot going through her mind. Or he might be so turned on by the idea that you go on to have the best sex you have ever had as a couple.

Whatever he feels, you should start by telling him how much it means to you and that you're not an expert by any stretch of the imagination. Like him, you are a novice and you would both be feeling your way along. You are about to open up to him and commit to each other in a way that is more intimate than almost any other because you are revealing your innermost thoughts and trusting him with secrets that you might never have dared to share before. When you get him onside and at least get him to agree to try it out, be kind to each other and listen to what the other person is saying. There is no wrong or right way to do this; it is more about what feels good to both of you.

Start Slowly

You might experience feelings of guilt to start with, and this is quite understandable because all through your life you have been indoctrinated that your place in a male dominated society is to serve men. This might be especially true if you were raised in a religious home where anything outside the dictates of what is regarded as vanilla sex is denigrated as being taboo. Your guilt is just an indication of how well and how long women have been suppressed under male dominance.

However, there are two sides to this coin and as society changes around us because of the introduction of technology and its rapid pace, man's role within it changes too. Whereas men might have expected to have manual jobs and a clearly defined role that was physical and masterful, the need for such jobs is quickly disappearing. He finds himself floundering in a world where he is beginning to feel superfluous to requirements. He becomes unsure of his identity and who he really is. However, he might have been raised in a household where his father was the patriarch and anything that he could not understand was ridiculed or abhorred. So the man you meet now has been very well trained to stay within those parameters. To step outside of them would cause him immense guilt too. And he is used to seeing his mother playing the little woman at home. Add to this that he might be a university graduate who has progressed into a high-powered job where he is expected to take decisions which might even affect others' lives on a daily basis. He is constantly stressed, but gets on with the job at hand because that is what is expected of him. Since he was born, not only has his family drilled into him that he must be a man and provide for his family, and but films and media have contrived to push this fact home to him. But now everything around him is changing and he is left in a confused state of flux.

When we look at it like this, men are having just as hard a time as women in adapting to the new dictates and requirements of a civilization which is driven by technology and roles in general are changing out of recognition to those of just a few decades ago. Alongside that, sex is becoming more visible and vocal. People are beginning to break out of the closet and stand up for what they really want and be who they feel they are, instead of pretending to fit the standard one size fits all. Try and see yourself as a suffragette for women's rights and you are participating in actions that will rid women of any guilt and shame that may have been inculcated within them to keep them in their place. Communication with your partner is the key. You should both be there to help and support the other one on their journey. Do not try and launch into a fully blown S&D relationship. Take your time and get to

196

know what you and your partner enjoy. Liken it to learning to drive. You would not expect to get into the driver's seat and know immediately how to drive without making any mistakes along the way. It is a process that has to be learned like any other and the more information you can gather, the quicker the process is made and the more confident you will both become.

Your partner may feel much more comfortable if your dominance is combined seamlessly with romance. Ask him to make you feel like a lady again. Tell him you want him to write you love letters or poetry and recite them to you. Tell him you want to recapture the romance you used to feel. If your partner has expressed the sentiment that he will never be able to let you whip him, then you must find another route to your destination. It might take longer to arrive than you wanted it to but if you apply the right attention it will be well worth the wait. Even the greatest of studs who consider themselves sexual champions can be shocked when female dominance is first suggested to them. Instead, this might suggest that rather than being the open-minded liberal they thought themselves to be, they are encased within their own masculinity – or their idea of what a masculine man should be. Any thought of relinquishing this could fill them with a horror of their abrupt emasculation.

Imagine a male dominant having the roles reversed. How would he be likely to approach the subject of domination of his partner? Typically, he would not ask for permission or say that he would like it to be discussed before entering into the action. At best, he might ask his partner what she likes sexually, but quite often it is taken as read that the woman is enjoying whatever a confident dominant submits her to. In fact, even when she asks him to stop – or even begs him to – he may still assume that this is still part of the game and continue. She may well have to scream 'rape' before he puts the brakes on and comes to realize that she actually means what she says.

If you find yourself in a sexual relationship with a man like this, it may be what you prefer. However, if you want to be able to turn the tables, you have many tricks up your sleeve at your disposal. Your arsenal is the most powerful of all the sex tools. You may have to be more persuasive, but there is always a way to get a man to do as you wish. If he tries to insist on being the dominant partner, you must show him quite firmly that you are not agreeable to it. If he tries to force you, then delay enjoyment for him. Set him tasks to perform like cooking a meal for you. When he does something that pleases you, reward him. This might just be by giving him a very long sexy kiss. Dress for the part and laugh at the same time, don't be put off your stride if he tries to pull you towards him and take over your plans. Or you might just stroke his penis through his pants. Or you could put both hands inside his pants and squeeze his ass cheeks while you're kissing him. Try being rough in bed and you take the lead. Pull his hair while you are having sex. Initiate sex when you feel like it, not when he does, and deny him sex when he does. Brush up on where his erogenous zones are and try them all out to establish which is the most powerful to get his engine running.

Flirt with him. Flirting is such a potent aphrodisiac. Tell him what you want him to do to you. Have phone sex with him. Ring him at work and whisper very dirty things into his ear, especially when you can be sure that someone else is near to him and might overhear you speaking on his phone.

Buy him presents such as a cock ring and you put it on him. Buy him a chastity belt and insist he wears it. In bed, make sure you climb on top of him so that you can regulate the sex. When he is about to climax, climb off and say, "Not yet big boy. I'm not ready. You will have to please me a lot more than that." And then sit on his face and tell him to lick your pussy because it's getting far too wet. You regulate the timing until you make it excruciating for him and he begs you to let him come. Don't let him until you are ready. Make it the best night he has ever had. Make him bend over and try fucking him, maybe with a strap-on dildo you have bought or your own vibrator. Or perhaps with a finger at this stage.

When you have serviced him, tell him to get up and get you a glass of wine or cup of coffee. Say that you are only having a rest and you need more of him so that he can't go to sleep just yet. Ask him to rub your whole body down with oil and then offer your breast for him to suck. While he's doing that, keep telling him that he's a good boy and that he's doing a good job. He's really turning you on. Now tell him to rub your clitoris just the way you like it. There is only him that does it right because he's so good. He gives you it just the way you like it. Keep giving him a little bit at a time. Get on all fours and tell him to fuck you from the back. The way that you're introducing your dominance is very subtle. You're asking him to do things for you but then praising him and telling him that he's the stud. Intersperse this with normal requests such as could he get your phone for you because you can hardly walk after the seeing-to he's just given you. If he tries to mount you without being instructed to do so, tell him to get off you because you're in charge tonight and you want to save some for him so that you can go on for longer and give him what he deserves. If he tries to spank you, slap him and tell him that is not allowed. Bit by bit, you are taking his power away from him and before he knows it, he will be eating out of your hand. Remember always to assume the position on top during sex until he gets used to the idea that you are in charge.

As he becomes more and more used to the things you want to introduce, start bringing more things into it: gags, butt plugs, blindfold, hand-cuffs. Keep telling him that he is really turning you on and that you can't get enough of him. If he carries on you are going to suck his cock like he's never had it sucked before. When you do that, put a finger up his ass and with a finger on your other hand, gently squeeze his balls and stroke the part between his balls and his anus. This should turn him on so much that he is putty in your hands.

Keep the impetus going by reminding him the next morning how much you enjoyed yourself and then ask him to bring you breakfast in bed because you are so exhausted and you have to gather your strength so that you will be able to repeat it. Inch by inch, introduce him to new experiences and these should be interspersed with tasks you wish to delegate to him. If you haven't been able to get him to do the garden, for instance, promise him a night to remember if he makes a start on it immediately. Of course, you are using sex to get what you want. But why wouldn't you? You are both getting what you want and you not only get the house looking good, but you get to live out your fantasy of being a female dominant. If you're clever, he won't even be aware you're doing it. He will be very grateful for the marvelous sex life he's been gifted with.

Greet him when he returns from work wearing nothing but stockings, high heels, and a hat. Tell him you want him now and instruct him to strip off completely and fuck you over the kitchen table. Then tell him to order food and open wine and you lounge around on the sofa telling him to hurry up and come and satisfy you quick. I doubt that he'll refuse.

So from being in a partnership with a macho dominant man who you loved in all other respects, he is quickly growing into the completely ideal man you have been seeking all your life. You could also introduce your man to female dominant literature and films. How would he like to have a zany, erotic and exotic night out? Tell him that you have to dress up in fancy dress and that you are going to meet lots of wild and colorful people. Be upbeat and enthusiastic about it. After visiting such a place, he might find that he's had such an excellent time that he wants to go back.

Another way of playing out your dominance with a hitherto dominant man is to suggest cuckolding. Quite often this turns on a man who perceives himself as being macho. He enjoys seeing other men having a good time with his partner and being able to be present makes him feel complicit in the naughtiness. He might think because it is not within the realms of what is considered normal by society at large, that he is being naughty too. So this takes us back to when he was little again and is still a form of male submission. The woman is being fucked by another man right in front of him and he is actually giving his consent for her to do so. Who is in charge of the situation?

Equally, most men seem to be turned on by seeing two women together. If you are bisexual or even you could quite easily convince your partner to comply with our wishes that you have sex with other women as long as you allow him to watch. He is not allowed to have sex with her, and he might not be allowed to watch you either having sex with a man or another woman. However, he will be incredibly excited by the prospect of you telling him exactly what happened afterward and promises him that he is promised the night of his life afterwards because the whole experience makes you feel so horny. He should lap it up and be eating out of your hand – or pussy – on command before you know it.

There are so many degrees and differences within S&D, so many variations of what it constitutes, so much for you to explore. So it is going to take a lot of discussion between the two of you and a lot of experimentation. The frequency and intensity is something that you will not know when you first start. In fact, you might not even know where or how to start. The first place perhaps to explore is through the Internet, magazines, movies, and books. At the end of your research, you might decide that you want to start off softly, but then after doing the same thing repeatedly you want to go a little deeper and be more daring and adventurous. Like anything else, if you do something over and over without changing it at all, it is likely to become boring and predictable, so try to be open-minded to keep things fresh and exciting.

You could start by buying some sexy underwear. Images of female dommes are prevalent and easily obtained all over the Internet but no doubt you or your partner may have something in mind already. If you feel embarrassed about buying these in person, have a look for something online so that it can be sent to you discreetly. Even wearing sexy underwear under your work clothes can give your sex life a new lease. You don't have to build the dungeon in your basement immediately, as soon as you get agreement from your partner to try S&D out. Don't splash out on a load of expensive equipment to start with. You might find you've shelled out a month's salary on stuff you're never likely to use again. Use your imagination in as many areas that will improve your sex life as you can. Improvise with equipment. No one says you have to have metal handcuffs and a whip, especially not to begin with. What's wrong with a scarf and your hand, or even a belt if you both agree to it?

No doubt you are both going to feel self-conscious at first but once you start to grow in confidence this will disappear and you will be more ready to experiment with other things. Some couples might agree to visit a club and there are many around, some dedicated to male domination. Have a look and research what's near you. If you have to travel a good distance, make it a special event. If you do, try and see it for what it is: fun. You don't have to join in with anything but dress up and get in the spirit or otherwise you're liable to stand out like a sore thumb and look like tourists. Even observing others or talking to more experienced people will give you invaluable lessons that you might not be able to learn elsewhere. It will also make you identify with a group and help to satisfy those feelings that may be lurking in the recesses of your mind that you are abnormal. Don't take your parents with you in your head or this might never work. On the other hand, there's nothing wrong with feeling naughty. Sex can be naughty but nice.

At this stage, it is more about communication with your partner. Talk about what he would like to try out to persuade him that it might be well worth a try on some level. You can work out what to move onto as you go along. Ask him about what turns him on. What are his fetishes? Encourage him to open up to you. What you are aiming for is equality in the relationship, one that is

209

mutually satisfying so you tell him what you would like to try too. But don't try and rush things too quickly. Slowly, slowly catchy monkey.

If you do feel embarrassed at first, then try and go with the flow. Don't take any negative comments from your partner personally. If he asks you to do something differently, do not take it as a criticism but try and see this as part of the learning curve. If he puts you off, by commenting about something negatively while you are actually doing it, forbid him to speak during the session. Something like that could knock any confidence you were carefully building up right out of you. However, this is not to say that you shouldn't discuss it afterward. You want to learn from your experience and make them as pleasurable as you can for each other. Of course, you will make mistakes. We all do and you would be unnatural if you both did everything perfectly at first – either that, or very low in expectations. It is a game, and is to be enjoyed. You both make your own rules because it is your own personal game. You are devising it and making it up as you go along. Share the experience as fully as you can. It should be fun and if one of you is not enjoying it, you need to discuss openly why not and decide what you can do about it to ensure that both of you enjoy it in future.

However, do not be persuaded to do something which you do not wish to do, however heartfelt his pleas. If you start going against your natural instincts you are being controlled and manipulated, exactly the opposite to what you are hoping to achieve. Be steadfast. If you discuss it and you still feel the same at the end of the discussion, then say so and state your reasons why. And stick to your guns.

When you ask him questions or ask him to describe what he likes, don't just hear it but actively listen. If you do this, it should become a fuller and more comprehensive conversation and help you to give him exactly what he wants. If he does become overly critical of you during the session then remind him that he is there to please you. Of course, this would not apply if you are crossing the thresholds that you should have agreed before commencing the threshold. He is your servant and you must tell him that he is now going to be punished for his words. Make it part of the session. Try and force yourself to be dominant at first because you will grow into the person you are wishing to be if you act if out regularly.

Try and find a support group. This is not just for when you are starting out but can be seen as an ongoing group identity and offer support for whenever you flounder. You also get the chance to share what you've learned so far too with other women who might need the support just as much as you once did. Sometimes, it can help to talk to others who are in the same position as you. You can offer each other moral support and suggest solutions to any problems they are having but which you have managed to overcome. If you can't find any in your area, look for one online or start your own. Members of a peer group can suggest new things to try that have been successful for them so that it can help you to introduce new things that you might not have thought of or come across otherwise yourself. When you're feeling abnormal, peer group members can talk you through it and assure and convince you that whatever you choose to do within a loving relationship is perfectly acceptable. They are like any other friends you have but they add another dimension that your friends who are not part of an S&D relationship might not understand or be able to offer support around.

What if you are inexperienced when it comes to S&D and have been married or in a stable relationship when your partner suggests that he would like to try out this lifestyle? What should you do? Well, first of all, try not to be shocked at his proposal. He may have suppressed his longing for some time and be nervous or even afraid of suggesting such a thing to you for fear that you might see him differently or reject him. But he is still the same person who you loved before he told you of his desires. In fact, you should feel honored that he has finally found the courage to share his innermost desires. Ask him to tell you more about it and ask for more information on the subject. He may have had time to find out a lot of information while he has fought his inclinations and tried his best to suppress them. Be aware that he could have gone and paid for a professional domme to fulfill his fantasies but instead, he has chosen to confide in you because he loves you. You are his queen and he wants to make your love life more satisfying for both of you.

If you do feel disgust or shock, try and question why you do so. Are your reactions perhaps more to do with your own relationship with sex rather than his? Try and be open-minded and receiving. Don't push him away. Together you have found out that you can overcome most

214

obstacles in your path or at least find a way around them. There is no reason why this one should be any different and you might discover that it introduces something into your life that could be so wonderfully exhilarating and new. Be very honest and open about your thoughts. Perhaps he can help to dismiss any doubts you may feel, perhaps not, but you will never know unless you try. Respect him for his honesty and his strength. If you tell him that he should be ashamed at this stage, there might be no way of bridging the gap that you create by your harsh words about something which is very personal to him and part of who he is. It's natural that you should be filled with all kinds of unusual and maybe unwanted emotions when your husband/partner reveals his proposals. But rest assured, he is not a pervert or a freak or even abnormal, whatever your instincts guide your thoughts towards.

If you love each other, there is always room for negotiation to reach a compromise or agreement where both members of the partnership can be happy and flourish. But be warned, once you have enjoyed sex as a dominant woman or generally been dominant in your everyday lifestyle, it is always going to be difficult for you to revert to a life without it. Sex might be good in the future without your dominance being a feature of it but it will always seem like flat Champagne, however good it gets.

Different Ways of Being a Domme

Being in an S&D relationship is not all about sex exclusively. Men want to adopt the lifestyle in all sorts of degrees and this could incorporate financially, domestically, completely. Again, it's about negotiation and about what you both feel comfortable with but there are ways of subtly introducing S&D if you are not ready to introduce it in its entirety or neither of you wish to do so.

When this is first introduced to a woman by her partner, the woman often wonders where it has come from. Previously, she might have regarded her relationship with her partner to be perfectly acceptable and she was always satisfied with her sex life and her married life in general. But now her partner wants to introduce this new facet into their lives and she may be nervous about having the dynamics of their relationship tossed around and disturbed for potential destruction. What she must consider is that her partner has perhaps struggled with the concept for a long time and it has taken a lot of courage to introduce the idea to her.

Communication might open up to reveal that he is more interested in being controlled in other ways than sex. But it is likely that this proclivity probably stems from the relationship he developed with his mother or some other authority figure in his formative years. All he wanted to do then was to please that important woman who nurtured him and took care of him, and disciplined him when he needed it. Hopefully, she was firm but fair. He felt cared for and loved and that has sunken deep into his psyche and is an essential part of who he has become. It is only natural then that he would like to recreate this feeling with another significant woman in his life: you. Do not take his proclamations lightly. If you are shocked or alarmed, do your best to hide it. The very worst thing you can do is make him feel abnormal so that he shrinks back into himself and decides to satisfy his needs elsewhere.

Holding the power in a relationship might not involve all black leather and bondage. It can be much more subtle than that and it is much easier to introduce if this is the case. When you are in bed, ask him to do something for you and if he is reluctant to do so or even refuses, stroke his

218

penis, nibble his ear or perform whatever really turns him on. It doesn't have to be about performing actions that you might consider irregular or outlandish. This is more about timing and reminding him of how much pleasure you can give him if he treats you right. If you are confident about who you are and the sexual being that you are, this is an easy step to being able to get him to do whatever you want. Some women give their gift away far too easily and cannot understand why games must be played. However, if you don't value the marvelous gift you can bestow upon the chosen ones, why should anyone else value it? You have already proven to them that they don't have to prove themselves to you, that sex with you is on tap whenever they want it. Being permitted to have sex with you is like brandishing the metaphorical whip and it is surprisingly easy how men can quite rapidly change their minds with a bit of oral sex. But in order to receive, they must give, and you should make them work for it.

Since time immemorial, women have had the power to rule the world. And their partner. All you have to do is to grow into your power and make sure that you feel like the sex goddess you want him to see you as. Walk around as if you own the world and notice if men turn to look at you when you enter a room. Women do not have to be incredibly beautiful to attract attention; it is all about confidence. So start building it. And as your confidence grows, so will your partner's wish to fulfill your desires and receive favors from you. Sexual favors are not a joke, but it is something that has been portrayed as one as women's emancipation grows in society. Wanting equality can be a two-edged sword because it can so easily change the dynamics in the bedroom as well as the boardroom. You want your partner to see you as the most desirable woman in the world so act like one and the feeling will become real.

Try and discuss all aspects of being dominant to his submissive. How far does he wish to adopt this lifestyle? As you can see from above it doesn't have to take large leaps away from your normal sex lives. It can just be a redress of balance within the partnership. There are so many different ways you can incorporate female dominance and you might find that one runs on quite naturally from quite a tame start and develop into eye-popping raunchiness. You see it as a way to improve your life, which may or may not include domination. Your partner sees it as a way to get more sex and to fulfill his fantasies. Everyone's a winner, one way or another.

Various other suggestions that he might run past you might include one or more of the following:

Financial

This is often referred to as Findom and is more or less self-explanatory. Whether or not one or both of the couple works, the woman is in charge of the financial side of the household. Get his name taken off the joint bank account. Anything he earns must go into your bank account. This might involve her taking complete control of all finances and giving the man an allowance on which to manage despite him being the largest earner. Once you have complete financial control everything else should fall into place nicely. You can have a power of attorney so that you are allowed to sign for anything in place of your partner. You will pay all the bills from their joint income and make all financial decisions. You will decide how much you as a couple can spend on a social life, clothes, holidays and household bills.

Your partner receives an allowance decided upon by you, either weekly or monthly, but he must make a report to you of what he is spending his allowance on. Make him provide receipts and a weekly spreadsheet or list of expenditure. For anything he needs outside of his allowance he must make a special request to you and it is ultimately your decision whether or not he gets it.

Despite this sounding something he might wish to avoid at all costs, it does have benefits for both people in a partnership. At least when only one person is in charge of finances, there can be no misunderstanding about who has paid the bills or what is going out of the bank account. So there are no nasty surprises to be had because the female plans it all out. Be aware though, should anything go wrong, the blame comes to lie firmly at your door so don't see this as a license to spend, spend, spend on every frippery you see.

It also allows the male to step back and relinquish control, which he might welcome; especially should he have a stressful job. He might be involved in number crunching all day, every day at work, so the last thing he wants to do is come home and manage the household too. By giving his partner control, he is satisfying a basic need of being cared for and cherished.

Household Chores

Is there anybody out there who genuinely enjoys domestic chores? Cleaning the toilet? Washing the dishes? The endless vacuuming of carpets or mopping? By doing the household chores, your partner is showing you how much he cares for you and this might explain why so many dominant women enjoy and embrace such a lifestyle. Give him lots of encouragement and praise and cuddle him or promise him something sexy you are sure he will enjoy.

You might choose to incorporate this part of your dominant role into your S&D lifestyle in a big way and use it to humiliate him, thereby exploiting his submissive desires to the full. And how often, when your house needs cleaning, do others blame the woman for being a dirty slut? They might profess to be modern thinkers but it is when outmoded views like this escape them, you realize at once how deeply entrenched our society believes that the woman's place is in the kitchen. Well actually, it's not. But it can be in the bedroom sometimes.

When the S&D role play is more pronounced in the relationship, to encourage him to take a more active role in the housework, for instance, and in your strict dominant role, you might instruct him, in your most bitchy voice, to brush the toilet floor using a toothbrush because he seems to be neglecting the corners. Insist that he continues to clean it until it is up to your satisfaction. Quite often, because women have adopted the domestic role from the start of the relationship, she has grown used to doing things in her own inimitable style and her partner's efforts might not be quite up to par as far as she is concerned. Agreeing to incorporate the domestic side because of his submissive nature answers both of your needs perfectly. He gets to exploit his submissive side and you get the housework done to your satisfaction. It's not good for him to cut corners. If he is going to go along with this agreement, make him do a good job otherwise what's the point of it. He might be getting something from it – but it's in his own head only – and what's in it for you. Use your head - as well as other bits of you to get the best out of him.

Childcare

If you have children, you already know how stressful this can be, especially if you work as well. Running them to school each day in peak hour traffic is no picnic and studies have shown that a mother's heart rate can rise significantly

226

during this journey. Add to that, that the kids are screaming for whatever they want at the moment and you have a pile of ironing to do after work. That is after you have called in at the supermarket to pick up whatever you're having for dinner and having to race around it at a breakneck speed so that you are there to pick up the kids in time again. How much easier would it be if you have a househusband at home who can relieve you of all this pressure? Even if he still works, or maybe works from home, he can still relieve you of the most onerous tasks while you have a relatively easy day at work, socializing with workmates and enjoying what you do.

Feeling challenged intellectually is something that stays at home moms can miss and don't realize how much their lives are going to change by having children. However, because of societal changes precipitated by technology and women's rise in status, their traditional roles are evolving into something totally different to those their mothers and grandmothers might have experienced. A domestic role reversal might be truly appreciated by the man of the family who welcomes a break from what he has been trained to comply with from birth. Being at home with the children releases him to explore his feminine, softer side and can be beneficial for the children. They learn to adapt to the new world that is evolving around them and trains them to live comfortably and easily within it. They also benefit from having a male role model feature prominently in their lives, and this is especially true of a man who is unafraid of showing his softer, feminine side. He also gains by getting to know his children better and being a much stronger influence in their upbringing and the shaping of their characters.

Different Measures of Success

Everyone is different, as you will soon discover when you start the journey of BDSM. Your partner may well be very different to anyone else you might have met or shared such a relationship within the past. What you are both exploring is how to meet in the middle and share common experiences from which you both benefit. Why would you protest against your partner wanting to please you? It is just a question of working out how that is best achieved. He might want to only take parts out of the lifestyle, which are not highly sexual. If he does wish to participate in sexual role-playing he may be selective in what he wishes to practice and you both have to communicate your needs to the other to discover what they want. It is always about mutual satisfaction.

First, establish what you ideally would want and then use that as your starting point. It will be highly unlikely if your partner agrees willingly and gladly to all of your suggestions immediately and without protest. If he is completely taken aback by what you are suggesting then try to convey how important it is to you and how you could introduce diluted forms of it. While he might be very adamant that he does not want to be involved in sexual domination, he might be quite willing for you to make all the major household decisions or those involving the children. This might be a good time to show him how much of a sexy woman you can be and where sexual favors could be very neatly introduced. With just a little persuasion, say stroking his penis, and giving him wet and penetrative kisses, he could easily change his mind or at least warm to the idea. Eventually, you might get him to the stage where he knows to battle against you is futile.

Whatever shape or form your relationship takes, it should be developed within a safe and caring relationship. Do you, for instance, want to be treated like his queen and worshipped? This might involve running you a nice relaxing bubble bath and washing your hair, after which he could gently towel you down and blow-dry your hair. Get him to do your nails while he's about it. So far, nothing overtly sexual has occurred, but then if you go onto have sex afterward, you might command him to give you a massage followed by shaving your pubes and then licking your pussy until you have an orgasm. When you're entirely satisfied and relaxed you can perhaps allow him to have sex with you but you choose the position and he has to obey. You might even allow him to come if you are feeling generous. Nothing unusual or untoward has happened. At least nothing you or most other people would consider outside the realms of a normal sexual relationship. He may or may not realize that you have already introduced an element of S&D into your relationship and that he didn't find it too unpalatable; he might even have enjoyed it immensely.

He doesn't have to be a total pushover either. You don't want him to end up as a total wimp do you? So again, careful discussion must be allowed to take place. Let him have his say. He might not want it public that he is your sex slave every weekend and that he is subjected to being whipped or having butt plugs inserted. Or that you insist he wears women's underwear to work everyday under his very formal business suits. Conversely, he might relish the fact that you are telling all your girlfriends what you get up to in private, especially if you can tell him truthfully that they are now all working on their partners to get the same treatment. When he sees them eying him up knowingly and admiringly, hopefully that is going to make him feel good and make him even more willing to cooperate.

Blend the treatment that you dole out so that even though you might be telling him he has a small penis, he knows that it can't be true because it makes you scream and beg for it to be rammed even harder. Make sure he knows that you love him even though you are verbally ridiculing him because that is part of the game. He has to know that you cherish him and that you are doing this because you wanted to share something extremely intimate and private with him.

Think back to when you first starting dating and how keen he was to make an impression on you and make you happy. He brought you flowers and gifts and opened doors for you. What happened? What's changed? You relaxed into a comfortable relationship and you started taking each other for granted. It works both ways too. Gradually, the light of romance dulls and the passion goes out of the relationship. If you're lucky, you decide to take matters into your hands and move the relationship up a notch so that you can relight the flame within you both again. To do this, go back to the early days of when you first met and remember how it made you feel when he made you feel special, and how good it made him feel too to see the look of love in your eyes, shining back at him. He probably misses those days too so it shouldn't be too difficult to get him to work with you to rekindle that passion. You can bring back those days when you couldn't get enough of each other's bodies, those days when you just wanted to cuddle up in bed and forget the rest of the world. And then life took over.

You probably never gave it a second thought about how much power you held over your partner then and how easy it was to get him to do what you wanted. You still have that power but perhaps he needs reminding of it. And perhaps you do too. You are a very sexual being and you need to be proud of that and make sure everyone else notices of the pride you have in yourself. Visit your hair salon and ask for a style that makes you smile and feel good about yourself when you come out. Buy yourself some new make-up; perhaps have a facial and a massage. Get some new clothes, nothing too tarty but something classy, which enhances your natural body shape and makes the most of what you've got. High shoes are always a turn on for men and make women feel sexy as soon as they slip into them.

Even if they do make you wince a little, you don't have to wear them for long or walk a marathon in them; have them on until you get the desired effect, which shouldn't take long.

Be thankful for your sensuality and your sexuality and make the most of it. You are a sexy woman who has the power to dominate men in whichever way she chooses. Make your partner's eyes pop open with anticipation and surprise. Make him remember what he saw in you in the first place. Make his heart race and get him to remember how much he wanted to please you then and how you want him to do the same for you now. You don't have to play the equivalent of the vampy female predator. Just be sure about who you are and what you want. Make men's heads turn. This doesn't mean you have to wear skimpy clothes or flaunt everything you have in the shop window. Sexiness is more about self assuredness and confidence; it's about being happy to be who you are because you like

235

yourself very, very much and know how much you have to offer the world. It's about being the best you that you can be. Tone flabby bodies up, hone dull brains, get off the sofa and do something that interests you. Who would be interested in a drab looking lump of lard who isn't interested in anything but TV? Would you? And when you have shaped yourself into someone you are proud to be, you actually need no one else to tell you how beautiful you are because you already know. And you know how much you can offer your partner if he complies and is willing to help you bring back the excitement into your relationship. If he isn't, then there is something seriously wrong and you need to work on it and start asking questions urgently.

Listen to the answers because whatever he might fob you off with will have a kernel of truth in it and there is usually a way that you can bring things back on track. And when you get there, don't ever forget how close you came to the edge. Make him realize how lucky he is to have you. He may no longer be exactly the man you wanted, nor the man who you first got together with, but if you work at it, he can come very close to it again or even better and you'll end up with a new improved version.

If you're still in the first stages of your relationship, then you should have no doubt about what I'm saying. This early in the relationship you should be heady with love and having wild nights of passion when you are both eager to please each other with your sexual prowess. Can you imagine it ever being any different? Well, it will be unless you always treat your relationship as being precious and nurture it every day. Sometimes that means that you have to lead your partner gently in a direction without him even realizing it's happening. You have a very powerful gift. Use it well and instead of losing it over time, learn how to cultivate it and use it to its best advantage and its fullest capacity.

Relationships inevitably change as time passes. They should grow deeper with each person developing a greater understanding and love for the other person. If you're lucky, this should evolve naturally, but there might be a bit of pushing and shoving along the way until the dominant party rises to the top. This should be done from a stance of loving and caring and it is important to retain that feeling, however explorations fare along the way. Within a loving partnership, it might become irrelevant that you are the dominant party and quite without anyone noticing over the years, it may evolve naturally. It's up to you as a couple how far this invades your lives together. Nothing is written in stone and if you do try something that you feel you will never be able to survive, stick with it. As long as you truly love your partner, there is nothing that your partnership cannot survive and you can always find a way through.

What is Your Role as the Dominant Woman?

If you have developed the right mindset then adopting your role of a dominant woman should not present much of a problem. It's all a matter of confidence and knowing your partner and his desires. However, even though you assume the role of dominant woman does not mean you have to deny that sometimes you might need support to make decisions too. You are a dominant woman, not a superhuman. The role of dominant woman should feel natural after a while but it doesn't necessarily demand that you deny your true self just that you have strong expectations of the way you are treated by others, especially your partner.

Nor does it mean that you should make your partner's life a misery. He wants to continue to respect you and adore you. You don't have to make him terrified to achieve his wish to serve you and make you happy. His primary wish is to make you happy and that springs from his love. Of course, there are degrees of sexuality to be discovered almost on a sliding scale. While some men want to be completely dominated in all spheres of their lives, others are more satisfied to be able to serve their partners so that it passes almost without notice by the outside world. While one man might want to be tied down and have to submit to pain which ranges from mild to excruciating, another man might consider this type of treatment way beyond the realms of what might turn him on. Just because you are the dominant person in the partnership does not make you responsible for deciding exactly what will and what will not happen. This should always be a joint decision. He may begin to depend on your authority and look for you to make all important decisions and you might appreciate this but sometimes it is going to be necessary for you to consult with him to help you find a way through difficult problems. Remember that you are his partner, not his mother, although it might sometimes feel to one or both of you that you are. Some men even end up calling their partner's mom by mistake or design, but the very fact that they do speaks volumes.

If you find that your partner actually wants to embrace a full S&D sexual relationship, then you might be so excited that everything happens spontaneously. Alternatively, you may have to give some thought about how to make sure that you both get something worthwhile out of it. Explain that you have not got much experience either and ask him how he wants to approach it. It might be that he wants you to dress up in leather and have the full domme regalia: high boots, leather Basque, stockings. You have to offer him something back that he wants so that he feels happy to participate in what might seem to be an outlandish demand at first. But if you listen carefully and take note of his wishes, then you don't have to be too open about how you will reward him. By him not knowing when, or if, he will be rewarded for his efforts might make it even more exciting an experience, one which he will be more willing to repeat. Do your research. A session might go like this:

He arrives home from work to find you in full domme gear. You are standing with a hand on your hip and your legs are splayed and your head tilting, a cruel and calculating look on your face.

"Where have you been roach?"

(Make time for him to take it all it and be prepared for his mouth to drop open in amazement.)

"I've been at work, you know where I've been. Wh…. What the hell is going on here?"

"Don't ask me questions, you little toad. Come in and shut the door. And for god's sake close your mouth. You look like a real cretin!"

(At this stage there might be total bemusement, even amusement, depending on how much you've discussed previously. At this stage, you are just feeling your way and finding out what feels comfortable, so you should both be prepared to feel a little silly at first getting into role.)

"And address me as Mistress, if you know what's good for you. Say it, say it now."

"I've been at work Mistress."

"Hurry up and come in. I want you to remove your clothes and go to the bathroom."

"Yes, Mistress."

"Call me when you are in the bathroom and completely naked."

When he calls make him wait for a while for you. If he leaves the bathroom, say something like,

"How dare you leave the bathroom without my order? And I heard you the first time. I hate it when you shout. I am not deaf. Now go back to the bathroom and wait there for me naked. And do not let me finding you sitting down. We'll see if there is anything we can do with that sad excuse for a cock."

"Yes, Mistress."

Let him wait for as long as you like and when you can't stand it any longer, go and join him. If he is standing up, go to join him. Take something long, maybe a wooden spoon. If he is standing up and his penis is flaccid, lift it up with the spoon.

"What do you call that sad excuse? It's laughable."

"It's my cock. Mistress."

"Sad. Don't let me see you getting an erection or there will be consequences. Do you understand?

"Yes."

"Yes, what roach?" Tap him lightly on the penis with the spoon.

"Yes, Mistress. Sorry, Mistress."

"Bend over. Hold onto the edge of the bath. I want to inspect you."

Pull his butt cheeks apart and stick your spoon into his anus about an inch.

"Oh you like that do you roach. Well, we had better stop that if you are enjoying it. We're not here for your enjoyment. You must get yourself ready to please your Mistress. Do you agree?"

"Yes, Mistress."

"Get into the shower now roach."

Run the shower on cold and make him stand there under it.

"Well clean yourself roach. Or do I have to hose you down in the garden?"

"No, Mistress."

Pass him some sort of brush, nail or a brush you might use to clean the bath or even toilet.

"Scrub roach. (Pause) Harder. We want all the crap off you if you are coming near me, don't we roach?"

"Yes, Mistress."

"Good, keep it up. You are pleasing your Mistress. Okay, you may get out now. Bend over so that I can inspect you again."

Again, part his cheeks and inspect his anus, sticking the spoon up a bit further and maybe moving it gently around. Smack his ass and tell him to go and stand in the bedroom and wait for you. Make him wait a little while; perhaps you could have a coffee while he's waiting. When you join him, if he is not standing up waiting, punish him by hitting his ass with a spoon. Try and get the bit where the fleshy part meets the back of the leg so that it doesn't leave marks or cause too much pain to start with. Then lie down on the bed and pull your pants/thong to one side and call him over to you.

"Come here roach, and get between my legs. I want you to lick my pussy until I tell you to stop."

Get him to do this until you are satisfied. When you are, tell him to go stand in the corner facing the wall and leave him there for a while. When you are ready, call him over and repeat the same exercise, as above. Have a little snooze if you feel tired.

"That was okay roach. Did you like it too?"

"Yes, Mistress."

"Perhaps I might give you a little treat roach. Would you like that?"

"Yes, Mistress, yes please."

Get into your favorite position for sex.

"Come and make me nice and wet roach. You know what I like."

When you are wet enough and ready for sex, say,

"Okay roach, your time for a little treat. Fuck me now."

Try not to let him come. You can achieve this by squeezing his penis or stopping him intermittently. You can just order him not to come until you say so but this might be for when you are more experienced. If he does climax when you have told him not to however, then you can punish him again.

"Well, that was okay considering the size of your cock. But I think you are going to need much more training. What do you think of that roach?"

"I am very grateful to you Mistress. I am here to serve you."

"Of course you are. Now go run me a bath with some nice bath oil in it."

Have him wash you down and offer up your tits to be massaged with oil and ask him to rub some between your legs. When you are ready, get out of the bath and go and make yourself comfortable on the bed telling him to follow you. Lie on the bed with your legs apart and your knees bent and put your hand between your legs and rub until it feel good.

"Oo, that needs shaving. I want you to shave my pubes roach. Go and fetch the things you're going to need. And do not keep me waiting or you will be severely punished."

When he has finished, instruct him to clear everything away and then come back and lick/fuck you again until you are satisfied. When you are satisfied, tell him it wasn't quite up to your standards so that you think you are going to have to punish him so that he will try harder next time. Tell him to get on all fours and put a dog collar on him with a lead. Lead him to the other side of the bed and secure the lead to something so that he can't just run off. Spank him either with your hand or with another tool, perhaps something that you can use as a paddle this time. Try and find out the optimum level of pain he can withstand but not too hard the first time.

"Stand up. Go into the bathroom. You need another cold shower before you sleep."

"No, please Mistress. Not so cold. And I am hungry and thirsty."

"How dare you! Get in there now. I am going to make you very sorry. Never disobey me again!"

Proceed to give him a cold shower and tell him to remain silent. After a while (don't leave it too long) get him out and paddle his ass for answering back and disobeying. Take hold of the lead and take him to the kitchen.

"Okay, roach. Make me a nice chicken club sandwich and some nice frothy coffee. And it had better be the way I like it. Or else."

After you have finished eating you can allow him something to eat.

"Oh yes, you're hungry and thirsty too aren't you roach?"

"Yes, Mistress."

"Okay, well I'm not all bad. Get Rover's water dish. I will allow you to clean it and fill it with water. Now I think there are some scraps of chicken left so put them in another bowl and put them next to the water on the floor. Okay, down boy. You may eat and drink now."

Give his lead a gentle jerk. When he has finished tell him to clear up and put things away.

"Okay, time to settle down for the night. Go and use the bathroom and then come and see me in the bedroom."

When he joins you in the bedroom, tell him to bend over and inspect his anus again before inserting a butt plug or something that can serve as one. Smack his ass and take him by the lead to a cushion at the side of the bed.

"Down boy. This is where you sleep now until I say otherwise. Down!" Tug on his lead to make him get down on the cushion. Throw a blanket over him and go about your business.

Obviously this is just a suggested scenario and, of course, you must adapt it as you see fit and so that you feel comfortable with it. Hopefully, you have remembered to discuss with your partner the things that both of you would like to do and you will grow into your role in your own fashion over time. Also, don't forget to refresh your minds with your safe word. If you break down into a fit of giggles at first, don't let it put you off. It should be fun too but hopefully you will learn to uphold your stern and dominant persona over time so that it becomes convincing.

When you have been doing this for a while in your sex life, you might notice that it spreads to other parts of your life, almost without either of you realizing. You might suddenly discover that you are now instructing him on what to do and he is not objecting; in fact, he seems to be relishing his diminished responsibility for taking decisions and handing everything over to you, his Mistress, the woman whom he worships and adores.

What is not to like for you? You get everything done to your standards around the house – this is his punishment and the way he earns your favor. Make the most of it. If you do need to consult him on anything, you can always make it sound as if you are doing him a favor by letting him make a decision for once. Encourage him to show his softer side. You hold all the power. You always have done but you are now learning how to use it to its utmost capacity.

Enjoy!

Thanks again for making it this far! I would very much appreciate an honest review of the book.

Thanks in advance,

Alex

Made in the USA
Las Vegas, NV
29 January 2022

42545067R00144